ADOLESCENCE AND PSYCHOANALYSIS

ADOLESCENCE AND PSYCHOANALYSIS

The Story and the History

edited by
Maja Perret-Catipovic and François Ladame

French text translated by
Philip Slotkin

Routledge
Taylor & Francis Group
LONDON AND NEW YORK

Chapter 2: "The Transformations of Puberty", by Sigmund Freud, reprinted by permission of Sigmund Freud Copyrights from *Three Essays on Sexuality* (1905d), *Standard Edition, 7*: 207–230.

Chapter 3: "Adolescence", by Anna Freud, reprinted by permission of Sigmund Freud Copyrights and of International Universities Press from *Psychoanalytic Study of the Child, Volume 13* (1958), pp. 255–278.

Chapter 4: "On Adolescence", by Jeanne Lampl-de Groot, reprinted by permission of International Universities Press from *Psychoanalytic Study of the Child, Volume 15* (1960), pp. 95–103.

Chapter 5: "The Second Individuation Process of Adolescence", by Peter Blos, reprinted by permission of International Universities Press from *Psychoanalytic Study of the Child, Volume 22* (1967), pp. 162–186.

Chapter 6: "A Note on the Crisis of Adolescence", by Evelyne Kestemberg, translated from the French by permission of Presses Universitaires de France from: *Revue Française de Psychanalyse, 44* (1980), 523–530.

Chapter 7: "The Central Masturbation Fantasy, the Final Sexual Organization, and Adolescence", by Moses Laufer, reprinted by permission of Yale University Press from *Psychoanalytic Study of the Child, Volume 31* (1976), pp. 297–316.

First published 1998 by Karnac Books Ltd.

2 Park Square, Milton Park, Abingdon, Oxfordshire OX14 4RN
52 Vanderbilt Avenue, New York, NY 10017

Routledge is an imprint of the Taylor & Francis Group, an informa business

First issued in hardback 2019

First published in French under the title, *Adolescence et psychanalyse: une histoire*, edited by Maja Perret-Catipovic and François Ladame. Lausanne: Delachaux et Niestlé, 1997, Collection "Textes de base en psychanalyse".

British Library Cataloguing in Publication Data

A C.I.P for this book is available from the British library

ISBN: 978-1-85575-199-6 (pbk)
ISBN: 978-0-367-32300-4 (hbk)

Edited, designed, and produced by Communication Crafts

CONTENTS

ABOUT THE EDITORS

MAJA PERRET-CATIPOVIC is a psychologist and psychotherapist. She is in charge of the Unit for Suicide Prevention and Research (Units for Adolescents and Young Adults, Department of Psychiatry, Geneva University Hospitals) and is Lecturer at the Faculty of Psychology, University of Geneva.

FRANÇOIS LADAME is a psychiatrist and psychoanalyst, former president of the Swiss Psychoanalytical Society. He is the Head of the Units for Adolescents and Young Adults, Department of Psychiatry, Geneva University Hospitals, and Professor at the Faculty of Medicine, University of Geneva.

PREFACE

The concern of psychoanalysts, psychiatrists, and psychologists with adolescence is of relatively recent origin. After the foundations had been laid by Freud (1905d), a few noteworthy but isolated publications appeared. A large-scale study of the "adolescent phenomenon" commenced only after the Second World War.

The current plethora of literature on the particular—or particularly dangerous—psychic disorders of the adolescent age has tended to distract attention from the specificity of the developmental process with its perils and potentialities. The fundamental texts presented here are intended to fill precisely this gap.

The psychoanalytic contributions presented in this book deal principally with specific aspects of psychic functioning and development in adolescence. Four of the ten texts are original papers that offer a conspectus of our present-day psychoanalytic understanding of the process of adolescence and its vicissitudes. The others have, since their original publication, been essential reading in the field of adolescent psychoanalysis.

The juxtaposition of all this material in a single volume is intended to provide a new working tool for all concerned with the psychoanalytic understanding of adolescence.

Geneva, October 1997

Translator's note

To avoid the repetition of clumsy constructions such as "he or she" and "his or her", the masculine pronoun and possessive adjective have been used throughout the newly translated material to refer to both sexes where relevant.

ADOLESCENCE AND PSYCHOANALYSIS

CHAPTER ONE

Adolescence and psychoanalysis: the story of the history

Maja Perret-Catipovic and François Ladame

Adolescence and psychoanalysis: both of these terms are the victims of their own success. The word "adolescent" was used in a disparaging sense at the end of the nineteenth century, and nowadays everything is readily dismissed as "adolescent". As for "psychoanalysis", the term has emerged from a circle of initiates into everyday—perhaps too everyday—parlance, where it now punctuates all forms of humanistic discourse. In view of their success, might these words not be said to have lost their meaning?

If we venture to treat the two terms as a couple, the story of their union is one whose beginning is never-ending. We shall attempt here to determine their origins in so far as they are known to us. Let us for the moment consider the two terms separately and define them as follows.

Adolescence is the psychic process that allows the changes of puberty to be integrated. It begins as soon as puberty is cathected by the child, sometimes even before it is experienced in the body. In some cases this cathexis—whether positive or negative—arises on the occasion of the first physical manifestations of the generative capacity, whereas in others it may commence before any physical changes are felt. The link between puberty and the process of adolescence is clear, although the two classes of phenomena cannot be equated (even in time).

It is less easy to grasp the point when adolescence ends. This difficulty is probably responsible for the air of vagueness surrounding the term "adolescence". Let us take it that adolescence concludes when the identificatory transformations inherent in the adolescent process culminate in the assumption of a stable and irreversible sexual identity. Furthermore, the new identifications must allow the internalization of the social code and the acquisition by the individual of a status of his own that supersedes parental protection. It must be emphasized that adolescence has an end. That end is normal when the transformations mentioned above succeed, but pathological if the process of adolescence is short-circuited, preventing the subject from developing autonomy of thought and appropriating the sexually mature male or female body. Such faulting may be glaringly evident (as in severe pathology) or more or less subtly masked by adaptive or mutilating defences.

What is *psychoanalysis*? It is at one and the same time a procedure for the investigation of the unconscious area of psychic life, a therapeutic method based on this investigation, and a theory of the functioning of the human psyche. This is the concise definition adopted by the Swiss Psychoanalytical Society, whose Constitution and Bylaws it heads. Regarding the first aspect, it may be added that what is to be investigated includes the unconscious meaning not only of a subject's words but also of his actions and imaginary activities. As to psychoanalytic treatment, it differs from other forms of psychotherapy by interpretation of the transference (and of the countertransference), wishes, and resistances, as well as by providing a specific and unvarying setting in which all these factors are given maximum scope to unfold.

Links between psychoanalysis and adolescence

Whereas the discovery of infantile sexuality is one of the cornerstones of psychoanalysis, it is sometimes forgotten that in the Freudian view psychosexual development is a biphasic process: one phase comes to an end with the temporary setting aside of the oedipal conflicts of infancy and the onset of the latency period, while a second commences with puberty; the latter is the decisive phase [*krisis* = decision] that will confer upon infantile sexual life its final, normal form (Freud, 1905d). Let us add that this final form may be normal or abnormal. For all are agreed that, whereas everything is prepared in childhood, everything falls into place in adolescence (Kestemberg, 1980, and Chapter 6 of this book).

Obvious as this is, adolescence has generally been—and to some extent still is—relegated to the background. Why should this be? The first reason is that the at the time scandalous acknowledgement of infantile sexuality probably contributed to the ousting of puberty from its central position. The fascination immediately aroused by this discovery gave rise to important theoretical and clinical advances and to the extension of the method of psychoanalytic treatment to children, through the work of Melanie Klein and of Anna Freud. The controversy between these two great ladies of child psychoanalysis, and subsequently between their followers, has kept this fascination alive to this day.

Another reason might be connected with the nature of the disorders classically deemed to be the province of psychoanalytic treatment, namely neurotic disorders. A so-called neurotic subject suffers primarily from unconscious conflicts between the world of his wishes, which naturally demand satisfaction, and the judging agency that is quick to condemn such aspirations. Moreover, in the universe of unconscious wishes, infantile sexuality reigns supreme.

However, the importance assigned to infantile sexuality may perhaps also have served as a "screen-concern" to distract attention from adolescent sexuality. The integration of sexuality, in its function as a foundation of the human psyche, was perhaps more acceptable when mediated by infantile sexuality—which was ultimately "innocent", whatever one might think about its "perverse polymorphism"—than a sexuality enshrined in the reality of the adult body, a sexuality now freely exercisable because no longer held in check by the prepubertal child's physical and psychosexual limitations. This disconcerting truth did not escape Aristotle, who wrote in his *Rhetoric*: "Young men have strong passions and tend to gratify them indiscriminately. Of the bodily desires, it is the sexual by which they are most swayed and in which they show absence of self-control."

The last twenty years have witnessed a rekindling of interest in adolescence and in the modifications of psychic functioning that must take place during this period of development. On the one hand, the thirst for knowledge inseparable from any genuine psychoanalytic thought is a natural encouragement to exploration on the boundaries of our known world; and, on the other, psychoanalysts have in the last quarter-century proved willing to treat an increasing number of subjects whose pathology is inconsistent with the classical definition of neurosis. Whereas these new visitors to our psychoanalytic couches or armchairs do still suffer from conflicts originating in the sphere of wishes, these conflicts spread their tentacles more widely, encroaching upon these patients' narcissism and their capacity to establish a positive self-representation and a continuous sense of being. This capacity is often unstable if not positively chaotic. Paradoxically, the fact of experiencing a desire for someone other than oneself—which is indispensable to adult human sexuality and affords prospects of libidinal satisfaction and narcissistic enrichment (as well as, admittedly, an inevitable risk of frustration)—becomes a threat to the integrity of the subject's own sense of existence if his ego foundations are too fragile. The area of conflict thus shifts from simply *having* (in the sense of possessing the object of desire) towards *being*: for how is the individual to preserve his sense of being, a coherent self-image, while at the same time acknowledging himself to be the subject of desire, the bearer of his own desires, and the object of the desired object's desires?

This takes us to the very heart of adolescence, and more precisely to certain *miscarriages* of the adolescent phase of development that are of interest to contemporary psychoanalysis because it deems them to lie at the root of the characteristic disorders of many of its patients.

The role of individual psychoanalysts in the evolution of adolescent psychoanalytic practice and theory

The Minutes of the Vienna Psychoanalytic Society give a good impression of the concerns of FREUD [1856–1939] and his colleagues during the period 1906 to 1918 (Nunberg & Federn, 1962, 1967, 1974, 1975). The major issues of adolescence—masturbation, sex education, suicide attempts—recur frequently in the discussions, even if these concerns do not ultimately lead to precise theories (Marty, 1996; Ouvry, 1996). The references to adolescent sexuality (with its potential for consummation) are always allusive or peripheral, and Freud's text on puberty and the associated psychic transformations (Freud, 1905d, and Chapter 2 of this book) was at the time the only clear contribution on the subject.

The history of psychoanalysis is equivocal as to the position assigned by Freud to adolescence. However, when doubts are still expressed today about the analysability of adolescents, it is well to remember that, according to the available clinical information (with which we are all familiar), many of Freud's female patients belonged in that age group; Dora, for example, was 18 years old. This historical point has often been stressed. But another important factor might be partly responsible for the uncertainty. In the early years of the twentieth century, in contrast to the present situation, the words *Adoleszenz* and *adoleszent* were very uncommon in German. These two terms do appear in the *Gesammelte Werke* (Freud's complete works in their original language), but much less frequently than *Pubertät* [puberty]. Apart from the fact that the word *Adoleszenz* was not in common use at the time, Freud's training was of course medical, and his early background was in neurology and paediatrics. The detour through these two specialities inevitably led him to respect terminological custom by preferring the words *Pubertät, Jugend,* and *Jugendliche* [puberty, youth, and the young] to *Adoleszenz* when referring to the phenomena of adolescence. The *Standard Edition* of Freud's works has perhaps compounded the problem because at the time of its publication the English words "puberty" and "adolescence" were not used in exactly the same senses as the equivalent German words. Yet one thing is certain: an attentive reading of Freud's works reveals the importance he assigned to this period and, in particular, to the psychic transformations of puberty, in regard to adult sexual life as a whole.

Following Freud's inaugural work on the transformations of puberty (1905d) and the discussions of the early Viennese psychoanalysts on the subject of adolescence, a number of investigative trails were blazed in the second generation, which was that of Freud's "first" pupils. One of those pupils was SIEGFRIED BERNFELD [1892–1953], who was particularly interested in the links between psychoanalysis and education. He worked hard to secure the integration of psychoanalytic theories in the pedagogics of his time. In 1912–13, Bernfeld had founded his own young people's movement, which was distinguished from others of its kind by, in particular, the integration of psychoanalytic ideas from Freud's *Three Essays* in the understanding of adolescence. From 1915 on, Bernfeld attended meetings of the Vienna Psychoanalytic Society on an unofficial basis, where he continued to develop his theses on "young people" and "youth" (see the above linguistic comments). An outstanding psychoanalytic contribution of his was the paper "Concerning a typical form of male puberty", which he read to the Society on 15 February 1922 (Bernfeld, 1923). Meanwhile, HELENE DEUTSCH [1884–1982] was concentrating on the development of girls (Deutsch, 1925).

Another member of this generation, AUGUST AICHHORN [1879–1949], made a prominent contribution to adolescent psychoanalysis. He was surely one of the first to emphasize the crucial function of a capacity for empathy with young people in distress. As early as in 1925, he published *Wayward Youth*, which earned him an international reputation. In this book he gives an account of his experience as an educator in two boarding-schools for young delinquents and orphans in Austria, illuminated by the psychoanalytic training upon which he had just embarked. His role remains central in the ongoing relations between the psychoanalytic movement and educational circles.

Several groups of psychoanalysts were thus working on the theme of adolescence during the inter-war years, but always within a theoretical perspective limited to educational applications, whether normal or therapeutic. Psychoanalysis gained acceptance as a form of treatment first for adults and later for children, but nothing was heard for many years about its applicability to adolescents. Perhaps the shock of the tragic death of HERMINE VON HUG-HELLMUTH [1882–1924], who was murdered by the 16-year-old nephew she had tried to "psychoanalyse", caused more emphasis to be placed on the perils than on the benefits of psychoanalysis during this period of life.

MELANIE KLEIN [1882–1960], who—together with Anna Freud and von Hug-Hellmuth—first cultivated the still virgin soil of childhood for psychoanalysis, hardly ever ventured into the field of adolescence. Apart from one short paper on puberty (Klein, 1922) and the chapter setting out her views on "The technique of analysis in puberty" (Klein, 1932), she made no further incursions into it. This position is ultimately in line with her understanding of psychic functioning and the way it should be approached and, indeed, treated. The fundamental importance assigned by Klein to the death drive from the moment of birth distracted attention from the fate of the libido during the process of sexual maturation, in which puberty is pivotal. For example, she describes the onset of menstruation in the girl as "the outward and visible sign that the interior of her body and the children contained there have been totally destroyed" (Klein, 1932). Kleinian thought is thus resolutely directed towards the most archaic levels of the psyche, which are deemed decisive for the future psychic organization. In her view, everything depends on the capacity of the infant to negotiate his—constitutional—aggression in his early object relations. Adolescence is systematically approached by comparison with childhood, and its problems are seen as a repetition of those of the infantile oedipal stage. Understandably, the Kleinian school does not regard the transformations of puberty as fundamentally mutative where psychic functioning is concerned. Psychic disorders of adolescent onset are understood as repetitions of the infantile, and no specificity is assigned to the different age categories except as regards therapeutic technique (word association or play). This is one of the roots of the controversy between Melanie Klein and Anna Freud.

ANNA FREUD [1895–1982] held that child psychoanalysis could not be equated with that of adults and developed theses in support of the specificity of the former. Similarly, when she turned her attention to adolescent psychoanalysis, she refused to amalgamate this group of patients with children and adults. The same is true of all analysts who accept the dualism of the drives and assign an essentially organizing (or sometimes disorganizing) function to sexuality. Following her father, Anna Freud maintained that the upsurge of drive energy at the time of puberty introduced an imbalance between the id and the ego and weakened the latter. This meant that adolescents had little tolerance of frustration and were impelled to seek immediate pleasure rather than substitutive, sublimatory satisfactions. Again, the anxiety connected with the weakening of the ego must cause the defences to become more rigid. In view of these particular features, classical analysis was contraindicated. By this position, Anna Freud was assigning a quite specific place to adolescent pathology, and, although this did not mean that she sought to treat adolescents by psychoanalysis, her work is a continuation of that of the friends of her youth who continued to take an interest in this period of life. She remained open to all the ideas and experiments emerging in adolescent psychoanalysis.

This position differs radically from that of DONALD WINNICOTT [1896–1971], which is clear if not defensible. He wrote:

> There exists one real cure for adolescence, and only one, . . . [It] belongs to the passage of time and to the gradual maturational processes; these together do in the end result in the emergence of the adult person. This process cannot be hurried or slowed up, though indeed it can be broken into and destroyed, or it can wither up from within, in psychiatric illness. [Winnicott, 1961]

Yet Winnicott refers in the same paper to the problems of the identity crisis, which may be manifested in suicide attempts or severe depression, while at the same time maintaining that "we meet the challenge rather than set out to cure what is essentially healthy". The harm done by such statements can readily be imagined. The fact that a renowned paediatrician and psychoanalyst classified suicide attempts and severe depression among tokens of health cannot but have made for the trivialization of adolescent psychic disorders and deprived many young patients of the appropriate care they urgently needed.

A change of perspective becomes evident at the end of the 1950s. JEANNE LAMPL-DE GROOT [1895–1987], a Dutch psychoanalyst who was a pupil of both Sigmund and Anna Freud and the latter's friend, maintained that it was not only possible but also necessary to analyse adolescents. She also pointed out that the resistances to embarking on such treatments might be due to the fact that the period of adolescence was not systematically analysed in adult treatments (including those of psychoanalysts-to-be). The paper reproduced in Chapter 4 (Lampl-de Groot, 1960) demonstrates the new trend then emerging and also undertakes a noteworthy discussion of the fate of narcissistic cathexes by way of considerations on the ego ideal, the ego, and the superego.

The paper published by ANNA FREUD in 1958 (cf. Chapter 3 of this book) offers an initial summary review of the ever-increasing number of psychoanalytic contributions on adolescence. It bears witness to this pivotal moment in the history of psychoanalysis and adolescence when psychoanalytic theory, applied psychoanalysis, and psychoanalytic therapy come together—especially as, at the time of its publication, Moses Laufer had become one of the most brilliant satellites in the firmament of Anna Freud's universe. The whole question of the analysability of adolescents was coming to be seen in an entirely new light through the early work of Laufer, conducted before the very eyes of Sigmund's daughter. From the very beginning of her psychoanalytic training, Anna Freud had shared the interest of her fellow-students—Aichhorn, Bernfeld, Erikson, and Hoffer—in the psychoanalytic understanding of adolescence, but had been reluctant to treat adolescents by psychoanalysis. She now watched Laufer's experiments with interest, unfailing encouragement, and support. It is probably because of Anna Freud's privileged relations with the friends of her youth and later with Laufer that, in her 1958 paper, she defended the possibility and necessity of offering adolescents psychoanalytic treatment, even if she herself never ventured to undertake such treatment or to advocate it at the Hampstead Clinic, which was devoted to child psychoanalysis.

The career of MOSES LAUFER, now one of the great figures in adolescent psychoanalysis, began in Canada, where he trained as a social worker. He then left for Israel to work with immigrant children affected by the war. This experience was the basis of his wish to embark on psychoanalytic training. With the encouragement of his then chief, who also advised him to contact Anna Freud, Laufer began his training as an adult psychoanalyst at the Institute in London. To earn a living, he took a job at a youth club in London's East End, an area where violence was rife among adolescents, who, in their despair and lack of prospects, were wreaking havoc all around. In parallel with his training at the Institute of Psycho-Analysis in London, Laufer was invited by Anna Freud to take part in the Wednesday afternoon seminars at the Hampstead Clinic. He now began training with her as a child psychoanalyst and was asked to talk about his work in the East End. Moved not only by the destitution and distress of the young people Laufer described but also by his manifest understanding of them, Anna Freud urged him to continue this activity while carrying on with his psychoanalytic training. She even encouraged him to accept for treatment a young patient from this disadvantaged district, whose situation Laufer had described in a Wednesday afternoon clinical presentation. Anna Freud later worked actively to secure the opening of an adolescent consultation centre away from the Hampstead Clinic. By a fortunate coincidence, she was approached by a wealthy Dutch industrialist called Van Leer, who wished to fund an aid project for children or adolescents. The outcome was the opening in 1961–62 of the Young People's Consultation Centre. Anna Freud at first encouraged her co-workers at the Hampstead Clinic to take part in the Centre's activities. Within two or three years, she was so convinced of the value of the Centre's work that it became an extension of the Hampstead Clinic for training in work with adolescents.

Shortly afterwards, however, Van Leer changed tack and decided to devote his fortune to supporting other kinds of projects. Deprived of its funding, the Young People's Consultation Centre survived with difficulty until the London Borough of Brent's Education Department agreed to accept financial responsibility for its activities, now carried on under the new name of the Brent Consultation Centre. Here, experienced psychoanalysts received young patients for consultation and assessment. Laufer's first treatments convinced Anna Freud how much classical psychoanalysis could offer seriously ill adolescents. She therefore overcame her initial reservations and even devoted part of the substantial subsidy provided by the Grant Foundation of New York for the survival of the Hampstead Clinic to the establishment of the Centre for Research into Adolescent Breakdown. Under the latter's banner, it became possible to offer several years of psychoanalytic treatment to about a dozen adolescents with severe pathology irrespective of the means of the patients or their families.

The therapeutic experience accumulated in these admittedly quite exceptional conditions by Moses Laufer, Eglé Laufer, and the group of psychoanalysts around them was to lead to an original psychoanalytic theory of the psychopathology of adolescence (cf. Chapter 7). In Laufer's model, the body occupies a specific position, whether or not the process of development takes a normal course. Pathology is expressed preferentially through the body, which is the prime target of destructive attacks. In adult psychic disorders, the same attacks may be made on thought. The aim of the process of development is the establishment of a fixed and irreversible sexual identity. Moreover, adolescence has an end, whether normal or otherwise. Psychopathology is modelled in terms of a breakdown in development, a deadlock, or a foreclosure, and not by reference to the traditional psychiatric nosography that is common currency in the case of adults (Laufer & Laufer, 1984). Furthermore, Laufer requires the psychoanalyst to adopt an unambiguous position on the issue of normality or pathology. For him, a psychoanalyst who establishes beyond doubt that there is a disorder in the development of an adolescent has no right to remain "neutral" but must clearly express his view of the risks incurred and the need for treatment. Conversely, in the case of transient disorders Laufer is much less demanding. Where proven pathology exists, he regards intensive psychoanalytic treatment (along classical lines) as clearly indicated.

Laufer has always been convinced of the need to encourage psychoanalytic societies to offer specific training in the field of adolescence, as well as of the importance of a forum in which to exchange experience for psychoanalysts working with adolescent patients. For this reason, together with one of us (F.L.), Philippe Gutton, Raymond Cahn, Robin Anderson, and a dozen or so other European psychoanalysts, he established the European Association for Adolescent Psychoanalysis [EAAP] in 1993.

In the United States, Peter Blos [1904–1997] was another analyst who deliberately concentrated in his writings on the study of adolescents, and in his clinical practice on the psychoanalytic treatment of adolescent patients. Observing that a theory of personality development based solely on the evolution of the libido was inadequate, and given his background in the American school, this author was to assign an important role to object-relations theory.

Blos divides adolescence into distinct developmental phases each with its own demands and conflicts (Blos, 1962). In particular, he distinguishes between preadolescence—characterized by an omnipresent fear of passivity and of submission to the archaic mother, accompanied by defensive idealization of the father—and the onset of adolescence itself—expressed through a qualitative change in the drives and the subordination of pregenitality to the working through of the Oedipus complex. Blos never ceased to emphasize that the Oedipus complex, in both its positive and its negative aspects, is not truly resolved until adolescence, having been temporarily set aside at the end of the infantile genital period. He was later to define adolescence as a "second individuation process" (Blos, 1967, and Chapter 5 of this book). Mahler had insisted on the need for the primary object to be internalized if separation from it is to be possible. Blos was to conclude that the essential task of adolescence is to disengage from this internalized object in order to be able to cathect new objects. He also assigned an important place to regression, which, in his view, is not merely defensive but constitutes an essential factor in the process of psychic development. He laid stress, too, on the importance of the father throughout the preoedipal period in helping the child emerge from the primitive dyad. This pre-oedipal father may give rise to significant complications in adolescence, in the form of a fixation to his grandiosity, with all the resulting risks of homosexual development and obstruction of the constitution of the adult ego ideal (Blos, 1984).

Let us now return to Europe, and more particularly France, where Pierre Mâle and Evelyne Kestemberg paved the way for the future flowering of psychoanalytic thought on adolescence. For many of our French colleagues, PIERRE MÂLE [1900–1976] remains the "father" of the French school of adolescent psychoanalysis, because he emphasized that adolescence did not merely mark the end of the infantile phase but also constituted an origin, and hence a revolution (Mâle, 1982). Gutton, among many others, acknowledges him as a master. In 1962, EVELYNE KESTEMBERG [1918–1989] published a paper on the vicissitudes of identification in adolescence, in which she linked the problem complex of the object, which centres on identification, with that of narcissism, which involves identity (Kestemberg, 1962). Throughout her life she continued to develop and enrich her ideas on this link, as the text we have chosen to reproduce here shows (see Chapter 6). The link between narcissism and the craving for the object remains paramount for many French psychoanalysts concerned with adolescence. This is true particularly of PHILIPPE JEAMMET, who may be placed in direct line of descent from Evelyne Kestemberg. Like her, he emphasizes the role of the fragility of adolescent patients' narcissistic foundations and the need to allow for this in the therapeutic indications. Jeammet has made outstanding contributions to the dissemination of a psychoanalytic view of adolescent disorders among psychiatrists and psychologists, initially in France, as head of the adolescent and young adult psychiatry department at the International Hospital of Paris University, and later in the world at large, through his presidency of the International Society for Adolescent Psychiatry [ISAP]. On the scientific level, his writings on anorexia nervosa, on the psychopathology of adolescence in general (Jeammet, 1990), and on dependence-related disorders in particular, as well as on the individual psychoanalytic psychodrama, are of fundamental importance.

Unlike Mâle and Kestemberg, PIERA AULAGNIER [1923–1990] never worked in the field of adolescence. Nevertheless, this emblematic figure in contemporary French psychoanalysis does in our view have a legitimate place here. On the one hand, Aulagnier greatly influenced the thought of present-day theorists of adolescence (Gutton and Ladame in particular), while, on the other, she was the author of a pioneering paper that illustrates and conceptualizes in exemplary fashion the difficulties inherent in acquiring true adolescent autonomy of thought (Aulagnier, 1984). On the basis of her knowledge of adult psychosis, she always laid stress on the autonomy of thought, which for her was an acquisition of adolescence that was essential to the constitution of the ego in the sense of the individual's psychic being. This point was taken up and developed by Cahn and Gutton, both of whom link the aspect of appropriation of the sexually mature male or female body (a point particularly emphasized by Laufer) to that of thought and its liberation from "external"—that is, parental—control.

Following the opening of a public-sector adolescent consultation and treatment centre in Geneva in 1973, lines of communication were gradually established between those working in the field in Switzerland, London, and Paris, in particular.

A new phase in the history of the links between psychoanalysis and adolescence was ushered in by the foundation of the journal *Adolescence* in 1983. It involved the formation around Gutton and one of the present authors (F.L.) of a group of psychoanalysts and practitioners engaged in the treatment of adolescents and in the conceptualization of specific aspects of the developmental process. This six-monthly journal of psychoanalysis, psychopathology, and humanities soon became established in the French-speaking countries as the principal channel for the transmission of psychoanalytic thought on adolescence and information on clinical psychoanalysis with adolescents.

In his research at the University of Paris and later at Aix-en-Provence University, PHILIPPE GUTTON came to distinguish two separate periods in adolescence, namely the explosive "pubertal" period when the psychic topography bursts asunder, giving free rein to incestuous and parricidal frenzy, and the healing "*adolescens*", characterized in particular by the formation of the adult superego and ego ideal (Gutton, 1991, 1996). These two periods are closely interwoven and do not constitute sequential phases. If they are defused, pathology ensues. The healing period is based on the establishment of original procedures that did not exist before puberty; hence the importance assigned to the transformations of the superego and the establishment of ideals (see Chapter 8).

The psychoanalytic understanding of adolescent psychosis is due mainly to RAYMOND CAHN. A member of the core group associated with the journal *Adolescence* from the beginning, he had established a day hospital for psychotic adolescents in Paris in 1972. Through his daily contacts with these patients and the team looking after them, Cahn was able to develop ideas on the theory and practice of the therapeutic institution, on the widened transference (extending to the institution and the team as a whole), on transitionality with reference to adolescents, and on the possibility of a psychoanalytic interpretation of the situation arising in such a setting (Cahn, 1991a). These ideas paved the way for this author's interest in the process of becoming-a-subject[1] and its vicissitudes (Cahn, 1991b, and Chapter 9 of this book).

Conclusion

The first dalliance between adolescence and psychoanalysis dates back to the very origins of the latter. Yet the history of their union is one of never-ending beginning. Psychoanalysis is conceivable only in terms of its three aspects: as theory, as a procedure for the investigation of the unconscious area of psychic life, and as a method of treatment. Adolescent psychoanalysis limped along for many years. The possibility of treating adolescents by psychoanalysis was disregarded until the end of the 1950s, perhaps because of the murder of von Hug-Hellmuth.

Fortunately, psychoanalysts such as Laufer in the United Kingdom and Blos in the United States did not allow themselves to be held back at the border and opened the way to genuine psychoanalytic work with adolescents. In the wake of their pioneering work, a number of adolescent consultation centres have been set up, such as the Geneva centre established in 1973 by one of the present authors (F.L.). Lines of communication for psychoanalytic ideas on adolescence have been organized (associations, journals, and congresses). One substantial problem remains to be solved: that of training for adolescent psychoanalysis. Not a single component society of the International Psychoanalytical Association [IPA] in Europe currently offers a training programme in adolescent psychoanalysis that is not amalgamated with training in child or adult psychoanalysis. The training function is, as a result, delegated to the various schools of psychotherapy. Even if psychoanalytically oriented, these cannot provide training in psychoanalysis. It is as if the idea of a genuine union between psychoanalysis and adoles-

[1]*Translator's note*: See Chapter 9, p. 149, note 1.

cence, notwithstanding its long history, still represented a danger and would therefore be conceivable only if the specificity of one or other of the partners were sacrificed.

The development of psychoanalysis in Latin America gives cause for hope. The psychoanalytic institutes of the IPA's component societies there have long offered training courses in adolescent psychoanalysis separate from those for child psychoanalysis, even if both are run by the same "department". This is all the more gratifying in view of the powerful influence of Kleinian thought in Latin America—proving that factional disputes are muted and give way to creative and dynamic innovation when our patients' interests are the prime object of our concern. May this example be a lesson to us.

CHAPTER TWO

The transformations of puberty

Sigmund Freud

With the arrival of puberty, changes set in which are destined to give infantile sexual life its final, normal shape. The sexual instinct has hitherto been predominantly auto-erotic; it now finds a sexual object. Its activity has hitherto been derived from a number of separate instincts and erotogenic zones, which, independently of one another, have pursued a certain sort of pleasure as their sole sexual aim. Now, however, a new sexual aim appears, and all the component instincts combine to attain it, while the erotogenic zones become subordinated to the primacy of the genital zone.[1] Since the new sexual aim assigns very different functions to the two sexes, their sexual development now diverges greatly. That of males is the more straightforward and the more understandable, while that of females actually enters upon a kind of involution. A normal sexual life is only assured by an exact

[1] [Footnote added 1915:] The schematic picture which I have given in the text aims at emphasizing differences. I have already shown above the extent to which infantile sexuality, owing to its choice of object and to the development of the phallic phase, approximates to the final sexual organization. [See also below.]

convergence of the affectionate current and the sensual current both being directed towards the sexual object and sexual aim. (The former, the affectionate current, comprises what remains over of the infantile efflorescence of sexuality.)[2] It is like the completion of a tunnel which has been driven through a hill from both directions.

The new sexual aim in men consists in the discharge of the sexual products. The earlier one, the attainment of pleasure, is by no means alien to it; on the contrary, the highest degree of pleasure is attached to this final act of the sexual process. The sexual instinct is now subordinated to the reproductive function; it becomes, so to say, altruistic. If this transformation is to succeed, the original dispositions and all the other characteristics of the instincts must be taken into account in the process. Just as on any other occasion on which the organism should by rights make new combinations and adjustments leading to complicated mechanisms, here too there are possibilities of pathological disorders if these new arrangements are not carried out. Every pathological disorder of sexual life is rightly to be regarded as an inhibition in development.

1. *The primacy of the genital zones and fore-pleasure*

The starting-point and the final aim of the process which I have described are clearly visible. The intermediate steps are still in many ways obscure to us. We shall have to leave more than one of them as an unsolved riddle.

The most striking of the processes at puberty has been picked upon as constituting its essence: the manifest growth of the external genitalia. (The latency period of childhood is, on the other hand, characterized by a relative cessation of their growth.) In the meantime the development of the internal genitalia has advanced far enough for them to be able to discharge the sexual products or, as the case may be, to bring about the formation of a new living organism. Thus a highly complicated apparatus has been made ready and awaits the moment of being put into operation.

[2] [This sentence was added in 1920.]

This apparatus is to be set in motion by stimuli, and observation shows us that stimuli can impinge on it from three directions: from the external world by means of the excitation of the erotogenic zones with which we are already familiar, from the organic interior by ways which we have still to explore, and from mental life, which is itself a storehouse for external impressions and a receiving-post for internal excitations. All three kinds of stimuli produce the same effect, namely a condition described as "sexual excitement", which shows itself by two sorts of indication, mental and somatic. The mental indications consist in a peculiar feeling of tension of an extremely compelling character; and among the numerous somatic ones are first and foremost a number of changes in the genitals, which have the obvious sense of being preparations for the sexual act—the erection of the male organ and the lubrication of the vagina.

Sexual tension

The fact that sexual excitement possesses the character of tension raises a problem the solution of which is no less difficult than it would be important in helping us to understand the sexual processes. In spite of all the differences of opinion that reign on the subject among psychologists, I must insist that a feeling of tension necessarily involves unpleasure. What seems to me decisive is the fact that a feeling of this kind is accompanied by an impulsion to make a change in the psychological situation, that it operates in an urgent way which is wholly alien to the nature of the feeling of pleasure. If, however, the tension of sexual excitement is counted as an unpleasurable feeling, we are at once brought up against the fact that it is also undoubtedly felt as pleasurable. In every case in which tension is produced by sexual processes it is accompanied by pleasure; even in the preparatory changes in the genitals a feeling of satisfaction of some kind is plainly to be observed. How, then, are this unpleasurable tension and this feeling of pleasure to be reconciled?

Everything relating to the problem of pleasure and unpleasure touches upon one of the sorest spots of present-day psychology. It will be my aim to learn as much as possible from the circumstances of the instance with which we are at present dealing, but I shall avoid any approach to the problem as a whole.[3]

Let us begin by casting a glance at the way in which the erotogenic zones fit themselves into the new arrangement. They have to play an important part in introducing sexual excitation. The eye is perhaps the zone most remote from the sexual object, but it is the one which, in the situation of wooing an object, is liable to be the most frequently stimulated by the particular quality of excitation whose cause, when it occurs in a sexual object, we describe as beauty. (For the same reason the merits of a sexual object are described as "attractions".) This stimulation is on the one hand already accompanied by pleasure, while on the other hand it leads to an increase of sexual excitement or produces it if it is not yet present. If the excitation now spreads to another erotogenic zone—to the hand, for instance, through tactile sensations—the effect is the same: a feeling of pleasure on the one side, which is quickly intensified by pleasure arising from the preparatory changes [in the genitals], and on the other side an increase of sexual tension, which soon passes over into the most obvious unpleasure if it cannot be met by a further accession of pleasure. Another instance will perhaps make this even clearer. If an erotogenic zone in a person who is not sexually excited (e.g. the skin of a woman's breast) is stimulated by touch, the contact produces a pleasurable feeling; but it is at the same time better calculated than anything to arouse a sexual excitation that demands an increase of pleasure. The problem is how it can come about that an experience of pleasure can give rise to a need for greater pleasure.

The mechanism of fore-pleasure

The part played in this by the erotogenic zones, however, is clear. What is true of one of them is true of all. They are all used to provide a certain amount of pleasure by being stimulated in the way appropriate to them. This pleasure then leads to an increase in

---

[3][Footnote added 1924:] I have made an attempt at solving this problem in the first part of my paper on *The Economic Problem of Masochism* (1924c).

tension which in its turn is responsible for producing the necessary motor energy for the conclusion of the sexual act. The penultimate stage of that act is once again the appropriate stimulation of an erotogenic zone (the genital zone itself, in the glans penis) by the appropriate object (the mucous membrane of the vagina); and from the pleasure yielded by this excitation the motor energy is obtained, this time by a reflex path, which brings about the discharge of the sexual substances. This last pleasure is the highest in intensity, and its mechanism differs from that of the earlier pleasure. It is brought about entirely by discharge: it is wholly a pleasure of satisfaction and with it the tension of the libido is for the time being extinguished.

This distinction between the one kind of pleasure due to the excitation of erotogenic zones and the other kind due to the discharge of the sexual substances deserves, I think, to be made more concrete by a difference in nomenclature. The former may be suitably described as "fore-pleasure" in contrast to the "end-pleasure" or pleasure of satisfaction derived from the sexual act. Fore-pleasure is thus the same pleasure that has already been produced, although on a smaller scale, by the infantile sexual instinct; end-pleasure is something new and is thus probably conditioned by circumstances that do not arise till puberty. The formula for the new function of the erotogenic zones runs therefore: they are used to make possible, through the medium of the fore-pleasure which can be derived from them (as it was during infantile life), the production of the greater pleasure of satisfaction.

I was able recently to throw light upon another instance, in a quite different department of mental life, of a slight feeling of pleasure similarly making possible the attainment of a greater resultant pleasure, and thus operating as an "incentive bonus". In the same connection I was also able to go more deeply into the nature of pleasure.[4]

---

[4] See my volume on *Jokes and their Relation to the Unconscious* which appeared in 1905 [near the end of Chapter IV]. The "fore-pleasure" attained by the technique of joking is used in order to liberate a greater pleasure derived from the removal of internal inhibitions. [In a later paper, on creative writing (1908e), Freud attributed a similar mechanism to aesthetic pleasure.]

Dangers of fore-pleasure

The connection between fore-pleasure and infantile sexual life is, however, made clearer by the pathogenic part which it can come to play. The attainment of the normal sexual aim can clearly be endangered by the mechanism in which fore-pleasure is involved. This danger arises if at any point in the preparatory sexual processes the fore-pleasure turns out to be too great and the element of tension too small. The motive for proceeding further with the sexual process then disappears, the whole path is cut short, and the preparatory act in question takes the place of the normal sexual aim. Experience has shown that the precondition for this damaging event is that the erotogenic zone concerned or the corresponding component instinct shall already during childhood have contributed an unusual amount of pleasure. If further factors then come into play, tending to bring about a fixation, a compulsion may easily arise in later life which resists the incorporation of this particular fore-pleasure into a new context. Such is in fact the mechanism of many perversions, which consist in a lingering over the preparatory acts of the sexual process.

This failure of the function of the sexual mechanism owing to fore-pleasure is best avoided if the primacy of the genitals too is adumbrated in childhood; and indeed things seem actually arranged to bring this about in the second half of childhood (from the age of eight to puberty). During these years the genital zones already behave in much the same way as in maturity; they become the seat of sensations of excitation and of preparatory changes whenever any pleasure is felt from the satisfaction of other erotogenic zones, though this result is still without a purpose—that is to say, contributes nothing to a continuation of the sexual process. Already in childhood, therefore, alongside of the pleasure of satisfaction there is a certain amount of sexual tension, although it is less constant and less in quantity. We can now understand why, in discussing the sources of sexuality, we were equally justified in saying of a given process that it was sexually satisfying or sexually exciting. It will be noticed that in the course of our enquiry we began by exaggerating the distinction between infantile and mature sexual life, and that we are now setting this right. Not only the deviations from normal sexual life but its normal form as well are determined by the infantile manifestations of sexuality.

2. *The problem of sexual excitation*

We remain in complete ignorance both of the origin and of the nature of the sexual tension which arises simultaneously with the pleasure when erotogenic zones are satisfied.[5] The most obvious explanation, that this tension arises in some way out of the pleasure itself, is not only extremely improbable in itself but becomes untenable when we consider that in connection with the greatest pleasure of all, that which accompanies the discharge of the sexual products, no tension is produced, but on the contrary all tension is removed. Thus pleasure and sexual tension can only be connected in an indirect manner.

Part played by the sexual substances

Apart from the fact that normally it is only the discharge of the sexual substances that brings sexual excitation to an end, there are other points of contact between sexual tension and the sexual products. In the case of a man living a continent life, the sexual apparatus, at varying intervals, which, however, are not ungoverned by rules, discharges the sexual substances during the night, to the accompaniment of a pleasurable feeling and in the course of a dream which hallucinates a sexual act. And in regard to this process (nocturnal emission) it is difficult to avoid the conclusion that

[5] It is a highly instructive fact that the German language in its use of the word *"Lust"* takes into account the part played by the preparatory sexual excitations which, as has been explained above, simultaneously produce an element of satisfaction and a contribution to sexual tension. *"Lust"* has two meanings, and is used to describe the sensation of sexual tension (*"Ich habe Lust"* = "I should like to", "I feel an impulse to") as well as the feeling of satisfaction.

the sexual tension, which succeeds in making use of the short cut of hallucination as a substitute for the act itself, is a function of the accumulation of semen in the vesicles containing the sexual products. Our experience in connection with the exhaustibility of the sexual mechanism argues in the same sense. If the store of semen is exhausted, not only is it impossible to carry out the sexual act, but the susceptibility of the erotogenic zones to stimulus ceases, and their appropriate excitation no longer gives rise to any pleasure. We thus learn incidentally that a certain degree of sexual tension is required even for the excitability of the erotogenic zones.

This would seem to lead to what is, if I am not mistaken, the fairly widespread hypothesis that the accumulation of the sexual substances creates and maintains sexual tension; the pressure of these products upon the walls of the vesicles containing them might be supposed to act as a stimulus upon a spinal centre, the condition of which would be perceived by higher centres and would then give rise in consciousness to the familiar sensation of tension. If the excitation of the erotogenic zones increases sexual tension, this could only come about on the supposition that the zones in question are in an anatomical connection that has already been laid down with these centres, that they increase the tonus of the excitation in them, and, if the sexual tension is sufficient, set the sexual act in motion or, if it is insufficient, stimulate the production of the sexual substances.[6]

The weakness of this theory, which we find accepted, for instance, in Krafft-Ebing's account of the sexual processes, lies in the fact that, having been designed to account for the sexual activity of adult males, it takes too little account of three sets of conditions which it should also be able to explain. These are the conditions in children, in females and in castrated males. In none of these three cases can there be any question of an accumulation of sexual products in the same sense as in males, and this makes a smooth application of the theory difficult. Nevertheless it may at once be admitted that it is possible to find means by which the theory may be made to cover these cases as well. In any case we are warned

[6] [This hypothesis had been discussed by Freud earlier: in Section III of his first paper on anxiety neurosis (1895b).]

not to lay more weight on the factor of the accumulation of the sexual products than it is able to bear.

Importance of the internal sexual organs

Observations on castrated males seem to show that sexual excitation can occur to a considerable degree independently of the production of the sexual substances. The operation of castration occasionally fails to bring about a limitation of libido, although such limitation, which provides the motive for the operation, is the usual outcome. Moreover, it has long been known that diseases which abolish the production of the masculine sex-cells leave the patient, though he is now sterile, with his libido and potency undamaged.[7] It is therefore by no means as astonishing as Rieger [1900] represents it to be that the loss of the masculine sex-glands in an adult may have no further effect upon his mental behaviour.[8] It is true that if castration is performed at a tender age, before puberty, it approximates in its effect to the aim of obliterating the sexual characters; but here too it is possible that what is in question is, besides the actual loss of the sex-glands, an inhibition (connected with that loss) in the development of other factors.

Chemical theory

Experiments in the removal of the sex-glands (testes and ovaries) of animals, and in the grafting into vertebrates of sex-glands from other individuals of the opposite sex,[9] have at last thrown a partial light on the origin of sexual excitation, and have at the same time

---

[7] [This sentence was added in 1920.]

[8] [The following sentence occurs at this point in editions before 1920, when it was omitted: "For the sex-glands do not constitute sexuality, and the observations on castrated males merely confirm what had been shown long before by removal of the ovaries—namely that it is impossible to obliterate the sexual characters by removing the sex-glands." Before 1920, too, the second half of the next sentence began: "but it seems that what is in question here is not the actual loss of the sex-glands but an inhibition. . . ."]

[9] Cf. Lipschütz's work (1919).

still further reduced the significance of a possible accumulation of cellular sexual products. It has become experimentally possible (E. Steinach) to transform a male into a female, and conversely a female into a male. In this process the psychosexual behaviour of the animal alters in accordance with the somatic sexual characters and simultaneously with them. It seems, however, that this sex-determining influence is not an attribute of that part of the sex-glands which gives rise to the specific sex-cells (spermatozoa and ovum) but of their interstitial tissue, upon which special emphasis is laid by being described in the literature as the "puberty-gland". It is quite possible that further investigation will show that this puberty-gland has normally a hermaphrodite disposition. If this were so, the theory of the bisexuality of the higher animals would be given anatomical foundation. It is already probable that the puberty-gland is not the only organ concerned with the production of sexual excitation and sexual characters. In any case, what we already know of the part played by the thyroid gland in sexuality fits in with this new biological discovery. It seems probable, then, that special chemical substances are produced in the interstitial portion of the sex-glands; these are then taken up in the blood stream and cause particular parts of the central nervous system to be charged with sexual tension. (We are already familiar with the fact that other toxic substances, introduced into the body from outside, can bring about a similar transformation of a toxic condition into a stimulus acting on a particular organ.) The question of how sexual excitation arises from the stimulation of erotogenic zones, when the central apparatus has been previously charged, and the question of what interplay arises in the course of these sexual processes between the effects of purely toxic stimuli and of physiological ones—none of this can be treated, even hypothetically, in the present state of our knowledge. It must suffice us to hold firmly to what is essential in this view of the sexual processes: the assumption that substances of a peculiar kind arise from the sexual metabolism.[10] For this apparently arbitrary supposition is

[10] [The whole of this paragraph as far as this point dates in its present form from 1920. In the first edition (1905) and the two subsequent ones the following

supported by a fact which has received little attention but deserves the closest consideration. The neuroses, which can be derived only from disturbances of sexual life, show the greatest clinical similarity to the phenomena of intoxication and abstinence that arise from the habitual use of toxic, pleasure-producing substances (alkaloids).

---

passage appears in its place: "The truth is that we can give no information on the nature of sexual excitation, especially since (having found that the importance of the sex-glands in this respect has been over-estimated) we are in the dark as to the organ or organs to which sexuality is attached. After the surprising discoveries of the important part played by the thyroid gland in sexuality, it is reasonable to suspect that we are still ignorant of the essential factors of sexuality. Anyone who feels the need of a provisional hypothesis to fill this wide gap in our knowledge may well take as his starting-point the powerful substances which have been found to be present in the thyroid gland and may proceed along some such lines as the following. It may be supposed that, as a result of an appropriate stimulation of erotogenic zones, or in other circumstances that are accompanied by an onset of sexual excitation, some substance that is disseminated generally throughout the organism becomes decomposed and the products of its decomposition give rise to a specific stimulus which acts on the reproductive organs or upon a spinal centre related to them. (We are already familiar with the fact that other toxic substances, introduced into the body from outside, can bring about a similar transformation of a toxic condition into a stimulus acting on a particular organ.) The question of what interplay arises in the course of the sexual processes between the effects of purely toxic stimuli and of physiological ones cannot be treated, even hypothetically, in the present state of our knowledge. I may add that I attach no importance to this particular hypothesis and should be ready to abandon it at once in favour of another, provided that its fundamental nature remained unchanged—that is, the emphasis which it lays upon sexual chemistry."—It is worth remarking how small a modification was made necessary in Freud's hypothesis by the discovery of the sex-hormones, which, indeed, he had anticipated not merely in 1905 but at least as early as in 1896, as may be seen from his two letters to Fliess, of March 1 and April 2 of that year (Freud, 1950a, Letters 42 and 44). He further insisted upon the importance of the chemical factor in his second paper on the part played by sexuality in the neuroses (1906a), published at about the same time as the first edition of the *Three Essays*.]

3. *The libido theory*[11]

The conceptual scaffolding which we have set up to help us in dealing with the psychical manifestations of sexual life tallies well with these hypotheses as to the chemical bases of sexual excitation. We have defined the concept of libido as a quantitatively variable force which could serve as a measure of processes and transformations occurring in the field of sexual excitation. We distinguish this libido in respect of its special origin from the energy which must be supposed to underlie mental processes in general, and we thus also attribute a *qualitative* character to it. In thus distinguishing between libidinal and other forms of psychical energy we are giving expression to the presumption that the sexual processes occurring in the organism are distinguished from the nutritive processes by a special chemistry. The analysis of the perversions and psychoneuroses has shown us that this sexual excitation is derived not from the so-called sexual parts alone, but from all the bodily organs. We thus reach the idea of a quantity of libido, to the mental representation of which we give the name of "ego-libido", and whose production, increase or diminution, distribution and displacement should afford us possibilities for explaining the psychosexual phenomena observed.

This ego-libido is, however, only conveniently accessible to analytic study when it has been put to the use of cathecting sexual objects, that is, when it has become object-libido. We can then perceive it concentrating upon objects,[12] becoming fixed upon them or abandoning them, moving from one object to another and, from these situations, directing the subject's sexual activity, which leads to the satisfaction, that is, to the partial and temporary extinction, of the libido. The psychoanalysis of what are termed transference neuroses (hysteria and obsessional neurosis) affords us a clear insight at this point.

---

[11] [This whole section, except for its last paragraph, dates from 1915. It is largely based on Freud's paper on narcissism (1914c).]

[12] [It is scarcely necessary to explain that here as elsewhere, in speaking of the libido concentrating on "objects", withdrawing from "objects", etc., Freud has in mind the mental presentations (*Vorstellungen*) of objects and not, of course, objects in the external world.]

We can follow the object-libido through still further vicissitudes. When it is withdrawn from objects, it is held in suspense in peculiar conditions of tension and is finally drawn back into the ego, so that it becomes ego-libido once again. In contrast to object-libido, we also describe ego-libido as "narcissistic" libido. From the vantage-point of psycho-analysis we can look across a frontier, which we may not pass, at the activities of narcissistic libido, and may form some idea of the relation between it and object-libido.[13] Narcissistic or ego-libido seems to be the great reservoir from which the object-cathexes are sent out and into which they are withdrawn once more; the narcissistic libidinal cathexis of the ego is the original state of things, realized in earliest childhood, and is merely covered by the later extrusions of libido, but in essentials persists behind them.

It should be the task of a libido theory of neurotic and psychotic disorders to express all the observed phenomena and inferred processes in terms of the economics of the libido. It is easy to guess that the vicissitudes of the ego-libido will have the major part to play in this connection, especially when it is a question of explaining the deeper psychotic disturbances. We are then faced by the difficulty that our method of research, psycho-analysis, for the moment affords us assured information only on the transformations that take place in the object-libido,[14] but is unable to make any immediate distinction between the ego-libido and the other forms of energy operating in the ego.[15]

For the present, therefore,[16] no further development of the libido theory is possible, except upon speculative lines. It would, however, be sacrificing all that we have gained hitherto from psy-

---

[13] [Footnote added 1924:] Since neuroses other than the transference neuroses have become to a greater extent accessible to psycho-analysis, this limitation has lost its earlier validity.

[14] [Footnote added 1924:] See the previous footnote.

[15] [Footnote added 1915:] Cf. my paper on narcissism (1914c). [Added 1920:] The term "narcissism" was not introduced, as I erroneously stated in that paper, by Näcke, but by Havelock Ellis. [Ellis himself subsequently (1928) discussed this point in detail and considered that the honours should be divided.]

[16] [This paragraph was added in 1920.]

cho-analytic observation, if we were to follow the example of C. G. Jung and water down the meaning of the concept of libido itself by equating it with psychical instinctual force in general. The distinguishing of the sexual instinctual impulses from the rest and the consequent restriction of the concept of libido to the former receives strong support from the assumption which I have already discussed that there is a special chemistry of the sexual function.

4. The differentiation between men and women

As we all know, it is not until puberty that the sharp distinction is established between the masculine and feminine characters. From that time on, this contrast has a more decisive influence than any other upon the shaping of human life. It is true that the masculine and feminine dispositions are already easily recognizable in childhood. The development of the inhibitions of sexuality (shame, disgust, pity, etc.) takes place in little girls earlier and in the face of less resistance than in boys; the tendency to sexual repression seems in general to be greater; and, where the component instincts of sexuality appear, they prefer the passive form. The auto-erotic activity of the erotogenic zones is, however, the same in both sexes, and owing to this uniformity there is no possibility of a distinction between the two sexes such as arises after puberty. So far as the auto-erotic and masturbatory manifestations of sexuality are concerned, we might lay it down that the sexuality of little girls is of a wholly masculine character. Indeed, if we were able to give a more definite connotation to the concepts of "masculine" and "feminine", it would even be possible to maintain that libido is invariably and necessarily of a masculine nature, whether it occurs in men or in women and irrespectively of whether its object is a man or a woman.[17]

---

[17] [Before 1924 the words from "libido" to the end of the sentence were printed in spaced type.—Footnote added 1915:] It is essential to understand clearly that the concepts of "masculine" and "feminine", whose meaning seems so unambiguous to ordinary people, are among the most confused that occur in science. It is possible to distinguish at least three uses. "Masculine"

Since I have become acquainted[18] with the notion of bisexuality I have regarded it as the decisive factor, and without taking bisexuality into account I think it would scarcely be possible to arrive at an understanding of the sexual manifestations that are actually to be observed in men and women.

Leading zones in men and women

Apart from this I have only the following to add. The leading erotogenic zone in female children is located at the clitoris, and is thus homologous to the masculine genital zone of the glans penis. All my experience concerning masturbation in little girls has related to the clitoris and not to the regions of the external genitalia that are important in later sexual functioning. I am even doubtful

---

and "feminine" are used sometimes in the sense of activity and passivity, sometimes in a biological, and sometimes, again, in a sociological sense. The first of these three meanings is the essential one and the most serviceable in psycho-analysis. When, for instance, libido was described in the text above as being "masculine", the word was being used in this sense, for an instinct is always active even when it has a passive aim in view. The second, or biological, meaning of "masculine" and "feminine" is the one whose applicability can be determined most easily. Here "masculine" and "feminine" are characterized by the presence of spermatozoa or ova respectively and by the functions proceeding from them. Activity and its concomitant phenomena (more powerful muscular development, aggressiveness, greater intensity of libido) are as a rule linked with biological masculinity but they are not necessarily so, for there are animal species in which these qualities are on the contrary assigned to the female. The third, or sociological, meaning receives its connotation from the observation of actually existing masculine and feminine individuals. Such observation shows that in human beings pure masculinity or femininity is not to be found either in a psychological or a biological sense. Every individual on the contrary displays a mixture of the character-traits belonging to his own and to the opposite sex; and he shows a combination of activity and passivity whether or not these last character-traits tally with his biological ones. [A later discussion of this point will be found in a footnote at the end of Chapter IV of *Civilization and its Discontents* (1930a).]

[18] [In 1905 only: "through Wilhelm Fliess".]

whether a female child can be led by the influence of seduction to anything other than clitoridal masturbation. If such a thing occurs, it is quite exceptional. The spontaneous discharges of sexual excitement which occur so often precisely in little girls are expressed in spasms of the clitoris. Frequent erections of that organ make it possible for girls to form a correct judgement, even without any instruction, of the sexual manifestations of the other sex: they merely transfer onto boys the sensations derived from their own sexual processes.

If we are to understand how a little girl turns into a woman, we must follow the further vicissitudes of this excitability of the clitoris. Puberty, which brings about so great an accession of libido in boys, is marked in girls by a fresh wave of *repression,* in which it is precisely clitoridal sexuality that is affected. What is thus overtaken by repression is a piece of masculine sexuality. The intensification of the brake upon sexuality brought about by pubertal repression in women serves as a stimulus to the libido in men and causes an increase of its activity. Along with this heightening of libido there is also an increase of sexual over-valuation which only emerges in full force in relation to a woman who holds herself back and who denies her sexuality. When at last the sexual act is permitted and the clitoris itself becomes excited, it still retains a function: the task, namely, of transmitting the excitation to the adjacent female sexual parts, just as—to use a simile—pine shavings can be kindled in order to set a log of harder wood on fire. Before this transference can be effected, a certain interval of time must often elapse, during which the young woman is anaesthetic. This anaesthesia may become permanent if the clitoridal zone refuses to abandon its excitability, an event for which the way is prepared precisely by an extensive activity of that zone in childhood. Anaesthesia in women, as is well known, is often only apparent and local. They are anaesthetic at the vaginal orifice but are by no means incapable of excitement originating in the clitoris or even in other zones. Alongside these erotogenic determinants of anaesthesia must also be set the psychical determinants, which equally arise from repression.

When erotogenic susceptibility to stimulation has been successfully transferred by a woman from the clitoris to the vaginal orifice, it implies that she has adopted a new leading zone for the purposes of her later sexual activity. A man, on the other hand, retains his leading zone unchanged from childhood. The fact that women change their leading erotogenic zone in this way, together with the wave of repression at puberty, which, as it were, puts aside their childish masculinity, are the chief determinants of the greater proneness of women to neurosis and especially to hysteria. These determinants, therefore, are intimately related to the essence of femininity.[19]

5. The finding of an object

The processes at puberty thus establish the primacy of the genital zones; and, in a man, the penis, which has now become capable of erection, presses forward insistently towards the new sexual aim—penetration into a cavity in the body which excites his genital zone. Simultaneously on the psychical side the process of finding an object, for which preparations have been made from earliest childhood, is completed. At a time at which the first beginnings of sexual satisfaction are still linked with the taking of nourishment, the sexual instinct has a sexual object outside the infant's own body in the shape of his mother's breast. It is only later that the instinct loses that object, just at the time, perhaps, when the child is able to form a total idea of the person to whom the organ that is giving him satisfaction belongs. As a rule the sexual instinct then becomes auto-erotic, and not until the period of latency has been passed through is the original relation restored. There are thus good reasons why a child sucking at his mother's breast has be-

---

[19] [The course of development of sexuality in women was further examined by Freud more particularly on four later occasions: in his case history of a homosexual woman (1920a), in his discussion of the consequences of the anatomical distinction between the sexes (1925j), in his paper on female sexuality (1931b), and in Lecture XXXIII of his *New Introductory Lectures* (1933a).]

come the prototype of every relation of love. The finding of an object is in fact a re-finding of it.[20]

The sexual object during early infancy

But even after sexual activity has become detached from the taking of nourishment, an important part of this first and most significant of all sexual relations is left over, which helps to prepare for the choice of an object and thus to restore the happiness that has been lost. All through the period of latency children learn to feel, for other people who help them in their helplessness and satisfy their needs, a love which is on the model of, and a continuation of, their relation as sucklings to their nursing mother. There may perhaps be an inclination to dispute the possibility of identifying a child's affection and esteem for those who look after him with sexual love. I think, however, that a closer psychological examination may make it possible to establish this identity beyond any doubt. A child's intercourse with anyone responsible for his care affords him an unending source of sexual excitation and satisfaction from his erotogenic zones. This is especially so since the person in charge of him, who, after all, is as a rule his mother, herself regards him with feelings that are derived from her own sexual life: she strokes him, kisses him, rocks him and quite clearly treats him as a substitute for a complete sexual object.[21] A mother would probably be horrified if she were made aware that all her marks of affection were rousing her child's sexual instinct and preparing for its later

---

[20] [Footnote added 1915:] Psycho-analysis informs us that there are two methods of finding an object. The first, described in the text, is the "anaclitic" or "attachment" one, based on attachment to early infantile prototypes. The second is the narcissistic one, which seeks for the subject's own ego and finds it again in other people. This latter method is of particularly great importance in cases where the outcome is a pathological one, but it is not relevant to the present context. [The point is elaborated in the later part of Section II of Freud's paper on narcissism (1914c).]

[21] Anyone who considers this "sacrilegious" may be recommended to read Havelock Ellis's views [1913, 18] on the relation between mother and child, which agree almost completely with mine.

intensity. She regards what she does as asexual, "pure" love, since, after all, she carefully avoids applying more excitations to the child's genitals than are unavoidable in nursery care. As we know, however, the sexual instinct is not aroused only by direct excitation of the genital zone. What we call affection will unfailingly show its effects one day on the genital zones as well. Moreover, if the mother understood more of the high importance of the part played by instincts in mental life as a whole—in all its ethical and psychical achievements—she would spare herself any self-reproaches even after her enlightenment. She is only fulfilling her task in teaching the child to love. After all, he is meant to grow up into a strong and capable person with vigorous sexual needs and to accomplish during his life all the things that human beings are urged to do by their instincts. It is true that an excess of parental affection does harm by causing precocious sexual maturity and also because, by spoiling the child, it makes him incapable in later life of temporarily doing without love or of being content with a smaller amount of it. One of the clearest indications that a child will later become neurotic is to be seen in an insatiable demand for his parents' affection. And on the other hand neuropathic parents, who are inclined as a rule to display excessive affection, are precisely those who are most likely by their caresses to arouse the child's disposition to neurotic illness.

Incidentally, this example shows that there are ways more direct than inheritance by which neurotic parents can hand their disorder on to their children.

Infantile anxiety

Children themselves behave from an early age as though their dependence on the people looking after them were in the nature of sexual love. Anxiety in children is originally nothing other than an expression of the fact that they are feeling the loss of the person they love. It is for this reason that they are frightened of every stranger. They are afraid in the dark because in the dark they cannot see the person they love; and their fear is soothed if they can take hold of that person's hand in the dark. To attribute to bogeys and blood-curdling stories told by nurses the responsibility for making children timid is to over-estimate their efficacy. The truth is merely that children who are inclined to be timid are affected by stories which would make no impression whatever upon others, and it is only children with a sexual instinct that is excessive or has developed prematurely or has become vociferous owing to too much petting who are inclined to be timid. In this respect a child, by turning his libido into anxiety when he cannot satisfy it, behaves like an adult. On the other hand an adult who has become neurotic owing to his libido being unsatisfied behaves in his anxiety like a child: he begins to be frightened when he is alone, that is to say when he is away from someone of whose love he had felt secure, and he seeks to assuage this fear by the most childish measures.[22]

The barrier against incest[23]

We see, therefore, that the parents' affection for their child may awaken his sexual instinct prematurely (i.e. before the somatic conditions of puberty are present) to such a degree that the mental excitation breaks through in an unmistakable fashion to the genital system. If, on the other hand, they are fortunate enough to avoid

---

[22] For this explanation of the origin of infantile anxiety I have to thank a three-year-old boy whom I once heard calling out of a dark room: "Auntie, speak to me! I'm frightened because it's so dark." His aunt answered him: "What good would that do? You can't see me." "That doesn't matter", replied the child, "if anyone speaks, it gets light." Thus what he was afraid of was not the dark, but the absence of someone he loved; and he could feel sure of being soothed as soon as he had evidence of that person's presence. [*Added* 1920:] One of the most important results of psycho-analytic research is this discovery that neurotic anxiety arises out of libido, that it is the product of a transformation of it, and that it is thus related to it in the same kind of way as vinegar is to wine. A further discussion of this problem will be found in my *Introductory Lectures on Psycho-Analysis* (1916–17), Lecture XXV, though even there it must be confessed, the question is not finally cleared up. [For Freud's latest views on the subject of anxiety see his *Inhibitions, Symptoms and Anxiety* (1926d) and his *New Introductory Lectures* (1933a), Chapter XXXII.]

[23] [This side-heading was omitted, probably by an oversight, from 1924 onwards.]

this, then their affection can perform its task of directing the child in his choice of a sexual object when he reaches maturity. No doubt the simplest course for the child would be to choose as his sexual objects the same persons whom, since his childhood, he has loved with what may be described as damped-down libido. But, by the postponing of sexual maturation, time has been gained in which the child can erect, among other restraints on sexuality, the barrier against incest, and can thus take up into himself the moral precepts which expressly exclude from his object-choice, as being blood-relations, the persons whom he has loved in his childhood. Respect for this barrier is essentially a cultural demand made by society. Society must defend itself against the danger that the interests which it needs for the establishment of higher social units may be swallowed up by the family; and for this reason, in the case of every individual, but in particular of adolescent boys, it seeks by all possible means to loosen their connection with their family—a connection which, in their childhood, is the only important one.[24]

It is in the world of ideas, however, that the choice of an object is accomplished at first; and the sexual life of maturing youth is almost entirely restricted to indulging, in phantasies, that is, in ideas that are not destined to be carried into effect.[25] In these phantasies the infantile tendencies invariably emerge once more, but

[24] [Footnote added 1915:] The barrier against incest is probably among the historical acquisitions of mankind, and, like other moral taboos, has no doubt already become established in many persons by organic inheritance. (Cf. my *Totem and Taboo*, 1912–13.) Psycho-analytic investigation shows, however, how intensely the individual struggles with the temptation to incest during his period of growth and how frequently the barrier is transgressed in phantasies and even in reality.—[Though this is its first published appearance, the "horror of incest" had been discussed by Freud on May 31, 1897 (Draft N in Freud, 1950a)—some months, that is, before his first revelation of the Oedipus complex. In that draft too he accounts for it on the ground that incest is "antisocial".]

[25] [Footnote added 1920:] The phantasies of the pubertal period have as their starting-point the infantile sexual researches that were abandoned in childhood. No doubt, too, they are also present before the end of the latency period. They may persist wholly, or to a great extent, unconsciously and for that reason it is often impossible to date them accurately. They are of great importance in the origin of many symptoms, since they precisely constitute

this time with intensified pressure from somatic sources. Among these tendencies the first place is taken with uniform frequency by the child's sexual impulses towards his parents, which are as a rule already differentiated owing to the attraction of the opposite sex—the son being drawn towards his mother and the daughter

---

preliminary stages of these symptoms and thus lay down the forms in which the repressed libidinal components find satisfaction. In the same way, they are the prototypes of the nocturnal phantasies which become conscious as dreams. Dreams are often nothing more than revivals of pubertal phantasies of this kind under the influence of, and in relation to, some stimulus left over from the waking life of the previous day (the "day's residues"). [See Chapter VII, Section I, of *The Interpretation of Dreams* (1900a); *S.E., 5,* 492 f.] Some among the sexual phantasies of the pubertal period are especially prominent, and are distinguished by their very general occurrence and by being to a great extent independent of individual experience. Such are the adolescent's phantasies of overhearing his parents in sexual intercourse, of having been seduced at an early age by someone he loves and of having been threatened with castration [cf. the discussion of "primal phantasies" in Lecture XXIII of Freud's *Introductory Lectures* (1916–17)]; such, too, are his phantasies of being in the womb, and even of experiences there, and the so-called "Family Romance", in which he reacts to the difference between his attitude towards his parents now and in his childhood. The close relations existing between these phantasies and myths has been demonstrated in the case of the last instance by Otto Rank (1909). [Cf. also Freud's own paper on "Family Romances" (1909c) and his long footnote to Section G of Part I of his case history of the "Rat Man" (1909d).]

It has justly been said that the Oedipus complex is the nuclear complex of the neuroses, and constitutes the essential part of their content. It represents the peak of infantile sexuality, which, through its after-effects, exercises a decisive influence on the sexuality of adults. Every new arrival on this planet is faced by the task of mastering the Oedipus complex; anyone who fails to do so falls a victim to neurosis. With the progress of psycho-analytic studies the importance of the Oedipus complex has became more and more clearly evident; its recognition has become the shibboleth that distinguishes the adherents of psycho-analysis from its opponents.

[*Added* 1924:] In another work (1924), Rank has traced attachment to the mother back to the prehistoric intra-uterine period and has thus indicated the biological foundation of the Oedipus complex. He differs from what has been said above, by deriving the barrier against incest from the traumatic effect of anxiety at birth. [See Chapter X of *Inhibitions, Symptoms and Anxiety* (1926d).]

towards her father.[26] At the same time as these plainly incestuous phantasies are overcome and repudiated, one of the most significant, but also one of the most painful, psychical achievements of the pubertal period is completed: detachment from parental authority, a process that alone makes possible the opposition, which is so important for the progress of civilisation, between the new generation and the old. At every stage in the course of development through which all human beings ought by rights to pass, a certain number are held back; so there are some who have never got over their parents' authority and have withdrawn their affection from them either very incompletely or not at all. They are mostly girls, who, to the delight of their parents, have persisted in all their childish love far beyond puberty. It is most instructive to find that it is precisely these girls who in their later marriage lack the capacity to give their husbands what is due to them; they make cold wives and remain sexually anaesthetic. We learn from this that sexual love and what appears to be non-sexual love for parents are fed from the same sources; the latter, that is to say, merely corresponds to an infantile fixation of the libido.

The closer one comes to the deeper disturbances of psychosexual development, the more unmistakably the importance of incestuous object-choice emerges. In psychoneurotics a large portion or the whole of their psychosexual activity in finding an object remains in the unconscious as a result of their repudiation of sexuality. Girls with an exaggerated need for affection and an equally exaggerated horror of the real demands made by sexual life have an irresistible temptation on the one hand to realize the ideal of asexual love in their lives and on the other hand to conceal their libido behind an affection which they can express without self-reproaches, by holding fast throughout their lives to their infantile fondness, revived at puberty, for their parents or brothers and sisters. Psychoanalysis has no difficulty in showing persons of this kind that they are *in love*, in the everyday sense of the word, with these blood-relations of theirs; for, with the help of their symptoms

---

[26] Cf. my remarks in *The Interpretation of Dreams* (1900a), on the inevitability of Fate in the fable of Oedipus [Chapter V, Section D; *S.E.*, *4*, 260 ff.].

and other manifestations of their illness, it traces their unconscious thoughts and translates them into conscious ones. In cases in which someone who has previously been healthy falls ill after an unhappy experience in love it is also possible to show with certainty that the mechanism of his illness consists in a turning-back of his libido onto those whom he preferred in his infancy.

After-effects of infantile object-choice

Even a person who has been fortunate enough to avoid an incestuous fixation of his libido does not entirely escape its influence. It often happens that a young man falls in love seriously for the first time with a mature woman, or a girl with an elderly man in a position of authority; this is clearly an echo of the phase of development that we have been discussing, since these figures are able to re-animate pictures of their mother or father.[27] There can be no doubt that every object-choice whatever is based, though less closely, on these prototypes. A man, especially, looks for someone who can represent his picture of his mother, as it has dominated his mind from his earliest childhood; and accordingly, if his mother is still alive, she may well resent this new version of herself and meet her with hostility. In view of the importance of a child's relations to his parents in determining his later choice of a sexual object, it can easily be understood that any disturbance of those relations will produce the gravest effects upon his adult sexual life. Jealousy in a lover is never without an infantile root or at least an infantile reinforcement. If there are quarrels between the parents or if their marriage is unhappy, the ground will be prepared in their children for the severest predisposition to a disturbance of sexual development or to a neurotic illness.

A child's affection for his parents is no doubt the most important infantile trace which, after being revived at puberty, points the way to his choice of an object; but it is not the only one. Other starting-points with the same early origin enable a man to develop

[27] [Footnote added 1920:] Cf. my paper *A Special Type of Choice of Object made by Men* (1910h).

more than one sexual line, based no less upon his childhood, and to lay down very various conditions for his object-choice.[28]

Prevention of inversion

One of the tasks implicit in object-choice is that it should find its way to the opposite sex. This, as we know, is not accomplished without a certain amount of fumbling. Often enough the first impulses after puberty go astray, though without any permanent harm resulting. Dessoir (1894) has justly remarked upon the regularity with which adolescent boys and girls form sentimental friendships with others of their own sex. No doubt the strongest force working against a permanent inversion of the sexual object is the attraction which the opposing sexual characters exercise upon one another. Nothing can be said within the framework of the present discussion to throw light upon it.[29] This factor is not in itself, however, sufficient to exclude inversion; there are no doubt a variety of other contributory factors. Chief among these is its authoritative prohibition by society. Where inversion is not regarded as a crime it will be found that it answers fully to the sexual inclinations of no small number of people. It may be presumed, in the next place, that in the case of men a childhood recollection of the affection shown them by their mother and others of the female sex who looked after them when they were children contributes powerfully to directing their choice towards women;[30] on the other

[28] [Footnote added 1915:] The innumerable peculiarities of the erotic life of human beings as well as the compulsive character of the process of falling in love itself are quite unintelligible except by reference back to childhood and as being residual effects of childhood.

[29] [Footnote added 1924:] This is the place at which to draw attention to Ferenczi's *Thalassa* (1924), a work which, though somewhat fanciful, is nevertheless of the greatest interest, and in which the sexual life of the higher animals is traced back to their biological evolution.

[30] [The rest of this sentence and the two following ones date from 1915. In the editions of 1905 and 1910 the following passage takes their place: "while in the case of girls, who in any case enter a period of repression at puberty, impulses of rivalry play a part in discouraging them from loving members of their own sex."]

hand their early experience of being deterred by their father from sexual activity and their competitive relation with him deflect them from their own sex. Both of these two factors apply equally to girls, whose sexual activity is particularly subject to the watchful guardianship of their mother. They thus acquire a hostile relation to their own sex which influences their object-choice decisively in what is regarded as the normal direction. The education of boys by male persons (by slaves, in antiquity) seems to encourage homosexuality. The frequency of inversion among the present-day aristocracy is made somewhat more intelligible by their employment of menservants, as well as by the fact that their mothers give less personal care to their children. In the case of some hysterics it is found that the early loss of one of their parents, whether by death, divorce or separation, with the result that the remaining parent absorbs the whole of the child's love, determines the sex of the person who is later to be chosen as a sexual object, and may thus open the way to permanent inversion.

CHAPTER THREE

Adolescence

Anna Freud

I. ADOLESCENCE IN THE PSYCHOANALYTIC THEORY

Introduction

I return to the subject of adolescence after an interval of twenty years. During this time much has happened in analytic work to throw added light on the problems concerned and to influence the conditions of life for young people, whether normal or abnormal. Nevertheless, in spite of partial advances, the position with regard to the analytic study of adolescence is not a happy one, and especially unsatisfactory when compared with that of early childhood. With the latter period, we feel sure of our ground, and in possession of a wealth of material and information which enables us to assume authority and apply analytic findings to the practical problems of upbringing. When it comes to adolescence, we feel hesitant and, accordingly, cannot satisfy the parents or educational workers who apply for help to us and to our knowledge. One can hear it said frequently that adolescence is a neglected period, a stepchild where analytic thinking is concerned.

These complaints, which come from two sides, from the parents as well as from the analytic workers themselves, seem to me to warrant closer study and investigation than they have received so far.

Adolescence in the psychoanalytic literature

The psychoanalytic study of adolescence began, as is well known, in 1905 with the relevant chapter of the *Three Essays on Sexuality*. Here, puberty was described as the time when the changes set in which give infantile sexual life its final shape. Subordination of the erotogenic zones to the primacy of the genital zone; the setting up of new sexual aims, different for males and females; and the finding of new sexual objects outside the family were listed as the main events. While this exposition explained many features of the adolescent process and behaviour which had been unexplained before, the newly developed notion of the existence of an infantile sex life could not but lower the significance of adolescence in the eyes of the investigators. Before the publication of the *Three Essays*, adolescence had derived major significance from its role as the beginning of sex life in the individual; after the discovery of an infantile sex life, the status of adolescence was reduced to that of a period of final transformations, a transition and bridge between the diffuse infantile and the genitally centred adult sexuality.

Seventeen years later, in 1922, Ernest Jones, London, published a paper on "Some Problems of Adolescence" which dwelt on a "correlation between adolescence and infancy" as its most distinctive point. Following the pronouncement in the *Three Essays* that the phase of development corresponding to the period between the ages of two and five must be regarded as an important precursor of the subsequent final organization, he showed in detail how "the individual recapitulates and expands in the second decennium of life the development he passed through during the first five years . . ." (p. 398). He ascribed the difference in "the circumstances in which the development takes place" but went as far as propounding "the general law . . . that adolescence recapitulates infancy, and that the precise way in which a given person will pass through the necessary stages of development in adolescence is to a very great extent determined by the form of his infantile development" (p. 399). In short: "these stages are passed through on different planes at the two periods of infancy and adolescence, but in very similar ways in the same individual" (p. 399).

Jones's important but isolated contribution to the problem coincided with a peak in the publications of Siegfried Bernfeld in Vienna, a true explorer of youth, who combined work as a clinical analyst and teacher of analysis with the unceasing study of adolescence in all its aspects of individual and group behaviour, reaction to social influences, sublimations, etc. His most significant addition to the analytic theory was the description of a specific kind of male adolescent development (1923), the so-called "protracted" type which extends far beyond the time limit normal for adolescent characteristics, and is conspicuous by "tendencies towards productivity whether artistic, literary or scientific, and by a strong bend towards idealistic aims and spiritual values . . .". As the solid background for his assumptions, Bernfeld published, in cooperation with W. Hoffer, a wealth of material consisting of self-observations of adolescents, their diaries, poetic productions, etc.

While Bernfeld accounted in this manner for the elaborations of the normal adolescent processes by the impact of internal frustrations and external, environmental pressures, August Aichhorn, also in Vienna, approached the problem from the angle of dissocial and criminal development. His work lay with those young people who answer to the same pressures with failure to adapt, faulty superego development and revolt against the community. His book *Wayward Youth* (1925) acquired world renown as the outstanding pioneering attempt to carry psychoanalytic knowledge into the difficult realm of the problems of the young offender.

Based on familiarity with S. Bernfeld's views, and intimately connected with A. Aichhorn's studies, I contributed in 1936 two papers under the titles "The Ego and the Id at Puberty" and "Instinctual Anxiety During Puberty". In my case, interest in the adolescent problems was derived from my concern with the struggles of the ego to master the tensions and pressures arising from the drive derivatives, struggles which lead in the normal case to character formation, in their pathological outcome to the formation of neurotic symptoms. I described this battle between ego and id as terminated by a first truce at the beginning of the latency period and breaking out once more with the first approach to puberty, when the distribution of forces inside the individual is upset by quantitative and qualitative changes in the drives. Threatened with anxiety by the drive development, the ego, as it has been formed in childhood, enters into a struggle for survival in which all the available methods of defence are brought into play and strained to the utmost. The results, that is the personality changes which are achieved, vary. Normally, the organization of ego and superego alter sufficiently to accommodate the new, mature forms of sexuality. In less favourable instances a rigid, immature ego succeeds in inhibiting or distorting sexual maturity; in some cases the id impulses succeed in creating utter confusion and chaos in what has been an orderly, socially directed ego during the latency period. I made the point that, more than any other time of life, adolescence with its typical conflicts provides the analyst with instructive pictures of the interplay and sequence of internal danger, anxiety, defence activity, transitory or permanent symptom formation, and mental breakdown.

Interest increased in the postwar years and brought a multitude of contributions, especially from the United States. Fortunately for the student of the subject, Leo A. Spiegel published in 1951 a lengthy "Review of Contributions to a Psychoanalytic Theory of Adolescence". Although his attempt to construct an integrated theory out of often widely divergent parts could hardly be successful, the paper serves a most useful purpose by abstracting, reviewing and classifying the material. He grouped the publications under headings such as:

"Classification of Phenomenology" (Bernfeld, Hartmann, Kris, and Loewenstein, Wittels)

"Object Relations" (Bernfeld, Buxbaum, H. Deutsch, Erikson, Fenichel, A. Freud, W. Hoffer, Jones, A. Katan-Angel, Landauer)

"Defense Mechanisms" (Bernfeld, H. Deutsch, Fenichel, A. Freud, Greenacre, E. Kris)

"Creativity" (Bernfeld, A. Freud)

"Sexual Activity" (Balint, Bernfeld, Buxbaum, H. Deutsch, Federn, Ferenczi, S. Freud, Lampl-de Groot)

"Aspects of Ego Functioning" (Fenichel, A. Freud, Harnik, Hoffer, Landauer)

"Treatment" (Aichhorn, K. R. Eissler, A. Freud, Gitelson, A. Katan, M. Klein, Landauer, A. Reich).

A detailed bibliography attached to the review contained altogether forty-one papers by thirty-four authors, covering apparently every theoretical, clinical, and technical aspect of the subject.

But in spite of this impressive list of contributors and contributions the dissatisfaction with our knowledge of the field remained unaltered, nor did our own, or the parents', confidence in our analytic skill with adolescent patients increase. There was now much published evidence to the contrary; nevertheless, adolescence remained, as it had been before, a stepchild in psychoanalytic theory.

Some difficulties of fact-finding concerning adolescence

There are, I believe, two different causes, which may, possibly, account for our bewilderment when faced with all the intricacies of the adolescent process.

When, in our capacity as analysts, we investigate mental states, we rely, basically, on two methods: either on the analysis of individuals in whom that particular state of mind is in action at the moment, or on the reconstruction of that state in analytic treatment undertaken at a later date. The results of these two procedures, used either singly or in combination with each other, have taught us all that we, as analysts, know about the developmental stages of the human mind.[1]

---

[1] It may be worth while to remind the reader in this connection that our knowledge of the mental processes of infancy has been derived from reconstructions in the analyses of adults and was merely confirmed and enlarged on later by analyses or observations carried out in childhood.

It happens that these two procedures, which have served us well for all other periods of life, prove less satisfactory and less productive of results when applied to adolescents.

1. *Reconstruction of adolescence in adult analysis*

As regards reconstruction, I am impressed how seldom in the treatment of my adult cases I succeed in reviving their adolescent experiences in full force. By that I do not mean to imply that adult patients have an amnesia for their adolescence which resembles in extent or in depth the amnesia for their early childhood. On the contrary, the memories of the events of the adolescent period are, normally, retained in consciousness and told to the analyst without apparent difficulty. Masturbation in preadolescence and adolescence, the first moves towards intercourse, etc., may even play a dominant part in the patients' conscious memories and, as we know well, are made use of to overlay and hide the repressed masturbation conflicts and the buried sexual activities of early childhood. Further, in the analyses of sexually inhibited men who deplore the loss of erective potency, it is fairly easy to recover the memories of the bodily practices carried out in adolescence—frequently very crude and cruel ones—which served them at that time to prevent erections, or to suppress them as soon as they occurred. On the other hand, these memories contain no more than the bare facts, happenings, and actions, divorced from the affects which accompanied them at the time. What we fail to recover, as a rule, is the atmosphere in which the adolescent lives, his anxieties, the height of elation or depth of despair, the quickly rising enthusiasms, the utter hopelessness, the burning—or at other times sterile—intellectual and philosophical preoccupations, the yearning for freedom, the sense of loneliness, the feeling of oppression by the parents, the impotent rages or active hates directed against the adult world, the erotic crushes—whether homosexually or heterosexually directed—the suicidal fantasies, etc. These are elusive mood swings, difficult to revive, which, unlike the affective states of infancy and early childhood, seem disinclined to re-emerge and be relived in connection with the person of the analyst.

If this impression, which I gathered from my own cases, should be confirmed by other analysts of adults, such a failure—or partial failure—to reconstruct adolescence might account for some of the gaps in our appraisal of the mental processes during this period.

2. *Analysis during adolescence*

When discussing in his "Review" the contributions dealing with the analytic therapy of adolescents, Spiegel (1951) deplored what seemed to him an undue pessimism on the part of some authors. He pointed to the need of adapting the analytic technique to the adolescent patients' particular situation and expressed surprise at the absence of explicit discussions of an introductory phase "analogous to the one used with children and delinquents".

Actually, since 1951, some further papers on the subject of technique appeared in print. Two of them dealt with the opening phase (Fraiberg, 1955; Noshpitz, 1957), a third with the terminal one (Adatto, 1958).

While these authors brought material to highlight the special technical difficulties encountered in the beginning and ending of the therapy, work on adolescents done in our Hampstead Child-Therapy Clinic emphasized special technical difficulties met with in the very centre of it, i.e. at the critical moment when preadolescence gives way to adolescence proper, when the revolt against the parents is anticipated in the transference and tends to lead to a break with the analyst, i.e. to abrupt and undesirable termination of treatment from the patient's side.

Thus, according to experience, special difficulties are encountered in the beginning, in the middle, and in connection with the end of treatment. Put in other words, this can only mean that the analytic treatment of adolescents is a hazardous venture from beginning to end, a venture in which the analyst has to meet resistances of unusual strength and variety. This is borne out by the comparison of adolescent with adult cases. In adult analysis we are used to handling the difficult technical situations with certain hysterical patients who cannot bear frustration in the transference and try to force the analyst to enact with them their revived love and hate feelings in an actual personal relationship. We are used to guarding against the obsessional patients' technique of isolating words from affect and of tempting us to interpret unconscious content while it is divorced from its emotional cathexis. We attempt to deal with the narcissistic withdrawal of the borderline schizophrenics, the projections of the paranoid patients who turn their analyst into the persecuting enemy, the destructive hopelessness of the depressed who claim disbelief in any positive outcome of the analytic effort; the acting-out tendencies and the lack of insight of the delinquent or psychopathic characters. But in the disturbances named above, we meet either the one or the other of these technical difficulties, and we can adapt the analytic technique to the resistance which is specific for the type of mental disorder. Not so in adolescence, where the patient may change rapidly from one of these emotional positions to the next, exhibiting them all simultaneously or in quick succession, leaving the analyst little time and scope to marshal his forces and change his handling of the case according to the changing need.

3. *Obstacles in the libido economy. Comparison with the states of mourning and unhappy love.*

Experience has taught us to take a serious view of such major and repeated inadequacies of the analytic technique. They cannot be explained away by individual characteristics of the patients under treatment nor by any accidental or environmental factors which run counter to it. Nor can they be overcome simply by increased effort, skill, and tact on the part of the analyst. They have to be taken as indications that something in the inner structure of the disturbances themselves differs markedly from the pattern of those illnesses for which the analytic technique has been devised originally and to which it is most frequently applied (Eissler, 1950). We have to gain insight into these divergences of pathology before we are in a position to revise our technique. Where the analyses of children, of delinquents, and of certain borderline states are concerned, this has happened already. What the analytic technique had to provide for in these cases were the immaturity and weakness of the patients' ego; their lower threshold for the toleration of frustration; and the lesser importance of verbalization with increased importance of action (acting out) for their mental economy. It remains to be pointed out what corresponding factors are characteristic for the adolescent disorders, i.e. to what specific inner situation of the patients our technique has to be adjusted to make adolescents more amenable to analytic treatment.

So far as I am concerned, I am impressed by a similarity between the responses of these young patients and those of two other well-known types of mental upset, namely the reactions to treatment during unhappy love affairs and during periods of mourning. In both these latter states there is much mental suffering and, as a rule, the urgent wish to be helped; in spite of this, neither state answers well to analytic therapy. Our theoretical explanation of this comparative intractability is the following: being in love as well as mourning are emotional states in which the individual's libido is engaged fully in relation to a real love object of the present, or of the most recent past, the mental pain being caused by the difficult task of withdrawing cathexis and giving up a position which holds out no further hope for return of love, that is, for satisfaction. While the individual is engaged in this struggle, insufficient libido is available to cathect the person of the analyst, or to flow back regressively and reinvest former objects and positions. Consequently, neither the transference events nor the past become meaningful enough to yield material for interpretation. The immediate object (of love, or of mourning) has to be given up before analytic therapy can become effective.

To my mind the libidinal position of the adolescent has much in common with the two states described above. The adolescent too is engaged in an emotional struggle, and moreover in one of extreme urgency and immediacy. His libido is on the point of detaching itself from the parents and of cathecting new objects. Some mourning for the objects of the past is inevitable; so are the "crushes", i.e. the happy or unhappy love affairs with adults outside the family, or with other adolescents, whether of the opposite or of the same sex; so is, further, a certain amount of narcissistic withdrawal which bridges the gap during periods when no external object is cathected. Whatever the libidinal solution at a given moment may be, it will always be a preoccupation with the present time and, as described above, with little or no libido left available for investment either in the past or in the analyst.

If this supposition as to the libido distribution in the adolescent personality can be accepted as a correct statement, it can serve to explain some of our young patients' behaviour in treatment, such as: their reluctance to cooperate; their lack of involvement in the therapy or in the relationship to the analyst; their battles for the reduction of weekly sessions; their unpunctuality; their missing of treatment sessions for the sake of outside activities; their sudden breaking off of treatment altogether. We learn here by contrast how much the continuity of the average adult analysis owes to the mere fact of the analyst being a highly cathected object, quite apart from the essential role played by the transference in the production of material.

There are, of course, those cases where the analyst himself becomes the new love object of the adolescent, i.e. the object of the "crush", a constellation which will heighten the young patient's keenness to be "treated". But apart from improved attendance and punctuality, this may mean merely that the analyst is brought up against another of the specific difficulties of the analyses of adolescents, namely the urgency of their needs, their intolerance for frustration and their tendency to treat whatever relationship evolves as a vehicle for wish fulfilment and not as a source of insight and enlightenment.

Under these conditions it is not surprising that besides analytic therapy many alternative forms of treatment for adolescents have been evolved and practised, such as manipulation of the environment, residential treatment, the setting up of therapeutic communities, etc. Valuable as these experimental approaches are from the practical point of view, they cannot, of course, be expected to contribute directly to our theoretical insight into the unconscious contents of the adolescent's mind, the structure of his typical disturbances, or into the details of the mental mechanisms by which these latter are maintained.

II. *CLINICAL APPLICATIONS*

What follows is an attempt to apply at least some of our hard-won insights to three of the most pressing problems concerning adolescence.

Is the adolescent upset inevitable?

There is, first, the ever recurrent question whether the adolescent upheaval is welcome and beneficial as such, whether it is necessary and, more than that, inevitable. On this point, psychoanalytic opinion is decisive and unanimous. The people in the child's family and school, who assess his state on the basis of behaviour, may deplore the adolescent upset which, to them, spells the loss of valuable qualities, of character stability, and of social adaptation. As analysts, who assess personalities from the structural point of view, we think otherwise. We know that the character structure of a child at the end of the latency period represents the outcome of long-drawn-out conflicts between id and ego forces. The inner balance achieved, although characteristic for each individual and precious to him, is preliminary only and precarious. It does not allow for the quantitative increase in drive activity, nor for the changes of drive quality which are both inseparable from puberty. Consequently, it has to be abandoned to allow adult sexuality to be integrated into the individual's personality. The so-called adolescent upheavals are no more than the external indications that such internal adjustments are in progress.

On the other hand, we all know individual children who as late as the ages of fourteen, fifteen, or sixteen show no such outer evidence of inner unrest. They remain, as they have been during the latency period, "good" children, wrapped up in their family relationships, considerate sons of their mothers, submissive to their fathers, in accord with the atmosphere, ideas, and ideals of their childhood background. Convenient as this may be, it signifies a delay of normal development and is, as such, a sign to be taken seriously. The first impression conveyed by these cases may be that of a quantitative deficiency of drive endowment, a suspicion which will usually prove unfounded. Analytic exploration reveals that this reluctance to "grow up" is derived not from the id but from the ego and superego aspects of the personality. These are children who have built up excessive defences against their drive activities and are now crippled by the results, which act as barriers against the normal maturational processes of phase development. They are, perhaps more than any others, in need of therapeutic help to remove the inner restrictions and clear the path for normal development, however "upsetting" the latter may prove to be.

Is the adolescent upset predictable?

A second question, which we are asked to answer frequently, concerns the problem whether the manner in which a given child will react in adolescence can be predicted from the characteristics of his early infantile or latency behaviour. Apart from the more general affirmative answer given by Ernest Jones (1922), only one among the authors named above has made clear and positive assertions in this respect. Siegfried Bernfeld (1923), when discussing his protracted type of male adolescence and its characteristics, established the links between this form of puberty and a specific type of infantile development based on the following three conditions: (a) that the frustration of infantile sex wishes has been shattering for the child's narcissism; (b) that the incestuous fixations to the parents have been of exceptional strength and have been maintained throughout the latency period; (c) that the superego has been established early, has been delineated sharply from the ego, and that the ideals contained in it are invested with narcissistic as well as with object libido.

Other and less precise answers to the same question are scattered through the literature. We find the opinion that, in the majority of cases, the manifestations of the adolescent process are not predictable since they depend almost wholly on quantitative relations, i.e. on the strength and suddenness of drive increase, the corresponding increase in anxiety causing all the rest of the upheaval.

I suggested in another place (1936) that adolescence brings about occasionally something in the nature of a spontaneous cure. This happens in children whose pregenital activities and characteristics remained dominant throughout latency until the increase in genital libido produces a welcome decrease in pregenitality. This latter occurrence, on the other hand, can be matched by a corresponding one which produces the opposite effect: where phallic characteristics have remained dominant during latency, the increase in genital libido produces the effect of an exaggerated and threatening aggressive masculinity.

It seems to be generally accepted that a strong fixation to the mother, dating not only from the oedipal but from the preoedipal attachment to her, renders adolescence especially difficult. This latter assertion, on the other hand, has to be correlated with two recent findings of a different nature which we owe to work done in our Hampstead Child-Therapy Clinic. One of these findings is derived from the study of orphaned children who were deprived of the relationship to a stable mother figure in their first years. This lack of a mother fixation, far from making adolescence easier, constitutes a real danger to the whole inner coherence of the personality during that period. In these cases adolescence is preceded frequently by a frantic search for a mother image; the internal possession and cathexis of such an image seems to be essential for the ensuing normal process of detaching libido from it for transfer to new objects, i.e. to sexual partners.

The second finding mentioned above is derived from the analyses of adolescent twins, in one case children whose twin relationship in infancy had been observed and recorded in minute detail (Burlingham, 1952). In their treatments it transpired that the "adolescent revolt" against the love objects of infancy demands the breaking of the tie to the twin in no lesser degree than the breaking of the tie to the mother. Since this libidinal (narcissistic as well as object-directed) cathexis of the twin is rooted in the same deep layer of the personality as the early attachment to the mother, its withdrawal is accompanied by an equal amount of structural upheaval, emotional upset, and resulting symptom formation. Where, on the other hand, the twin relationship survives the adolescent phase, we may expect to see a delay in the onset of maturity or a restrictive hardening of the character of the latency period similar to the instances mentioned above in which the childhood love for the parents withstands the onslaught of the adolescent phase.

To return to the initial question: it seems that we are able to foretell the adolescent reactions in certain specific and typical constellations but certainly not for all the individual variations of infantile personality structure. Our insight into typical developments will increase with the number of adolescents who undergo analysis.

Pathology in adolescence

This leaves us with a third problem which, to my mind, outweighs the preceding ones so far as clinical and theoretical significance are concerned. I refer to the difficulty in adolescent cases to draw the line between normality and pathology. As described above, adolescence constitutes by definition an interruption of peaceful growth which resembles in appearance a variety of other emotional upsets and structural upheavals.[2] The adolescent manifestations come close to symptom formation of the neurotic, psychotic, or dissocial order and merge almost imperceptibly into borderline states, initial, frustrated, or fully fledged forms of almost all the mental illnesses. Consequently, the differential diagnosis between the adolescent upsets and true pathology becomes a difficult task.

For the discussion of this diagnostic problem I leave most other authors in the field to speak for themselves and summarize my own impressions based on past and present clinical experience.

In 1936, when I approached the same subject from the aspect of the defences, I was concerned with the similarity between the adolescent and other emotional disturbances rather than with the differences between them. I described that adolescent upsets take on the appearance of a neurosis if the initial, pathogenic danger situation is located in the superego with the resulting anxiety being felt as guilt; that they resemble psychotic disturbances if the danger lies in the increased power of the id itself, which threatens the ego in its existence or integrity. Whether such an adolescent individual impresses us, then, as obsessional, phobic, hysterical, ascetic, schizoid, paranoid, suicidal, etc., will depend on the one hand on the quality and quantity of the id contents which beset the ego, on the other hand on the selection of defence mechanisms

---

[2] Adolescence, of course, is not the only time in life when alterations of a physiological nature cause disturbances of mental equilibrium. The same happens in later years in the climacterium; and recently, Grete L. Bibring (1959) has given a convincing description of similar damage to the equilibrium of mental forces during pregnancy.

which the latter employs. Since, in adolescence, impulses from all pregenital phases rise to the surface and defence mechanisms from all levels of crudity or complexity come into use, the pathological results—although identical in structure—are more varied and less stabilized than at other times of life.

Today it seems to me that this structural description needs to be amplified, not in the direction of the similarity of the adolescent to other disorders but in that of their specific nature. There is in their aetiology at least one additional element which may be regarded as exclusive to this period and characteristic for it: namely that the danger is felt to be located not only in the id impulses and fantasies but in the very existence of the love objects of the individual's oedipal and preoedipal past. The libidinal cathexis to them has been carried forward from the infantile phases, merely toned down or inhibited in aim during latency. Therefore the reawakened pregenital urges, or—worse still—the newly acquired genital ones, are in danger of making contact with them, lending a new and threatening reality to fantasies which had seemed extinct but are, in fact, merely under repression.[3] The anxieties which arise on these grounds are directed towards eliminating the infantile objects, i.e. towards breaking the tie with them. Anny Katan-Angel (1937) has discussed this type of defence, which aims above all at changing the persons and the scene of conflict, under the term of "removal". Such an attempt may succeed or fail, partially or totally. In any case, I agree with Anny Katan that its outcome will be decisive for the success or failure of the other, more familiar line of defensive measures which are directed against the impulses themselves.

A number of illustrations will serve to clarify the meaning of this assumption.

---

[3] An important clinical instance of this can be found in adolescent girls with anorexia nervosa. Here the infantile fantasies of oral impregnation receive added impetus from the new real possibilities of motherhood opened up by genital development. Consequently, the phobic measures adopted against the intake of food on the one hand and identification with the mother on the other hand are overemphasized to a degree which may lead to starvation.

(a) *Defence against the infantile object ties*

Defence by displacement of libido

There are many adolescents who deal with the anxiety aroused by the attachment to their infantile objects by the simple means of flight. Instead of permitting a process of gradual detachment from the parents to take place, they withdraw their libido from them suddenly and altogether. This leaves them with a passionate longing for partnership which they succeed in transferring to the environment outside the family. Here they adopt varying solutions. Libido may be transferred, more or less unchanged in form, to parent substitutes, provided that these new figures are diametrically opposed in every aspect (personal, social, cultural) to the original ones. Or the attachment may be made to so-called "leaders", usually persons in age between the adolescent's and the parents' generation, who represent ideals. Equally frequent are the passionate new ties to contemporaries, either of the same or of the opposite sex (i.e. homosexual or heterosexual friendships) and the attachments to adolescent groups (or "gangs"). Whichever of these typical solutions is chosen, the result makes the adolescent feel "free", and revel in a new precious sense of independence from the parents who are treated, then, with indifference bordering on callousness.

Although the direction taken by the libido in these instances is, in itself, on lines of normality, the suddenness of the change, the carefully observed contrast in object selection, and the overemphasis on the new allegiances mark it as defensive. It represents an all too hasty anticipation of normal growth rather than a normal developmental process.

It makes little further difference to the emotional situation whether the libidinal flight is followed by actual flight, i.e. whether the adolescent also "removes" himself bodily from his family. If not, he remains in the home in the attitude of a boarder, usually a very inconsiderate one so far as the older and younger family members are concerned.

On the other hand, the withdrawal of cathexis from the parents has most decisive consequences for the rest of the defensive processes. Once the infantile objects are stripped of their importance, the pregenital and genital impulses cease to be threatening to the same degree. Consequently, guilt and anxiety decrease, and the ego becomes more tolerant. Formerly repressed sexual and aggressive wishes rise to the surface and are acted on, the actions being taken outside the family in the wider environment. Whether this acting out will be on harmless, or idealistic, or dissocial, or even criminal lines will depend essentially on the new objects to which the adolescent has attached himself. Usually the ideals of the leader, of the adolescent group, or of the gang are taken over wholeheartedly and without criticism.

Adolescents of this type may be sent for treatment after their actions have brought them into conflict with their schools, their employers, or the law. As far as psychoanalytic therapy is concerned, they seem to offer little chance for the therapeutic alliance between analyst and patient without which the analytic technique cannot proceed. Any relationship to the analyst and, above all, the transference to him would revive the infantile attachments which have been discarded; therefore the adolescent remains unresponsive. Also, the escape from these attachments has suspended the feeling of internal conflict, at least temporarily; consequently, the adolescent does not feel in need of psychological help. A. Aichhorn had these points in mind when he maintained that adolescents of the dissocial and criminal type needed a long period of preparation and inner rearrangement before they could become amenable to analytic treatment. He maintained that the latter would be successful only if, during this preparation in a residential setting, the adolescent made a new transference of object love, reawakened his infantile attachments, internalized his conflicts once more, in short, became neurotic.

To try and analyse an adolescent in his phase of successful detachment from the past seems to be a venture doomed to failure.

Defence by reversal of affect

A second typical reaction to the same danger situation is, although less conspicuous outwardly, more ominous in nature inwardly.

Instead of displacing libido from the parents—or, more likely, after failing to do so—the adolescent ego may defend itself by turning the emotions felt towards them into their opposites. This changes love into hate, dependence into revolt, respect and admiration into contempt and derision. On the basis of such reversal of affect the adolescent imagines himself to be "free" but, unluckily for his peace of mind and sense of conflict, this conviction does not reach further than the conscious surface layer of his mind. For all deeper intents and purposes he remains as securely tied to the parental figures as he has been before; acting out remains within the family; and any alterations achieved by the defence turn out to his disadvantage. There are no positive pleasures to be derived from the reversed relationships, only suffering, felt as well as inflicted. There is no room for independence of action, or of growth; compulsive opposition to the parents proves as crippling in this respect as compulsive obedience to them can prove to be.[4] Since anxiety and guilt remain undiminished, constant reinforcement of defence is necessary. This is provided in the first place by two methods: denial (of positive feeling) and reaction formations (churlish, unsympathetic, contemptuous attitudes). The behavioural picture that emerges at this stage is that of an uncooperative and hostile adolescent.

Further pathological developments of this state of affairs are worth watching. The hostility and aggressiveness, which serve as a defence against object love in the beginning, soon become intolerable to the ego, are felt as threats, and are warded off in their own right. This may happen by means of projection; in that case the aggression is ascribed to the parents who, consequently, become the adolescent's main oppressors and persecutors. In the clinical picture this appears first as the adolescent's suspiciousness and, when the projections increase, as paranoid behaviour.

Conversely, the full hostility and aggression may be turned away from the objects and employed inwardly against the self. In these cases, the adolescents display intense depression and tendencies of self-abasement and self-injury, and develop, or even carry out, suicidal wishes.

During all stages of this process, personal suffering is great and the desire to be helped intense. This, in itself, is no guarantee that

[4] S. Ferenczi has pointed to this effect of "compulsive disobedience" many years ago.

the adolescent in question will submit to analytic therapy. He will certainly not do so if treatment is urged and initiated by the parents. Whenever this happens, he will consider analysis as their tool, extend his hostility or his suspicions to include the person of the analyst, and refuse cooperation. The chances are better if the adolescent himself decides to seek help and turns to analysis, as it were, in opposition to the parents' wishes. Even so, the alliance with the analyst may not be of long duration. As soon as a true transference develops and the positive infantile fantasies come into consciousness, the same reversal of affect tends to be repeated in the analytic setting. Rather than relive the whole turmoil of feelings with the analyst, many adolescent patients run away. They escape from their positive feelings, although it appears to the analyst that they break off treatment in an overwhelmingly strong negative transference.

Defence by withdrawal of libido to the self

To proceed in the direction of increasing pathology:

Withdrawal of libido from the parents, as it has been described above, does not, in itself, decide about its further use, or fate. If anxieties and inhibitions block the way towards new objects outside the family, the libido remains within the self. There, it may be employed to cathect the ego and superego, thereby inflating them. Clinically this means that ideas of grandeur will appear, fantasies of unlimited power over other human beings, or of major achievement and championship in one or more fields. Or, the suffering and persecuted ego of the adolescent may assume Christ-like proportions with corresponding fantasies of saving the world.

On the other hand, the cathexis may become attached to the adolescent's body only and give rise there to the hypochondriacal sensations and feelings of body changes that are well known clinically from initial stages of psychotic illness.

In either case analytic therapy is indicated as well as urgent. Treatment will dispel the appearance of severe abnormality if it reopens a path for the libido, either to flow backwards and recathect the original infantile objects or to flow forward, in the direction described above, to cathect less frightening substitutes in the environment.

What taxes the analyst's technical skill in these cases is the withdrawn state of the patient, i.e. the problem of establishing an initial relationship and transference. Once this is accomplished, the return from narcissistic withdrawal to object cathexis will relieve the patient, at least temporarily.

I believe, there are many cases where the analyst would be wise to be content with this partial success without urging further treatment. A further, and deeper, involvement in the transference may well arouse all the anxieties described above and, again, lead to abrupt termination of the analysis due to the adolescent's flight reaction.

Defence by regression

The greater the anxiety aroused by the object ties, the more elementary and primitive is the defence activity employed by the adolescent ego to escape them. Thus, at the extreme height of anxiety, the relations with the object world may be reduced to the emotional state known as "primary identification" with the objects. This solution with which we are familiar from psychotic illnesses implies regressive changes in all parts of the personality, i.e. in the ego organization as well as in the libido. The ego boundaries[5] are widened to embrace parts of the object together with the self. This creates in the adolescent surprising changes of qualities, attitudes, and even outward appearance. His allegiance to persons outside himself betrays itself in these alterations of his own personality (i.e. his identifications) rather than in an outflow of libido. Projections, together with these identifications, dominate the scene and create a give-and-take between the self and object which has repercussions on important ego functions. For example, the distinction between the external and internal world (i.e. reality testing) becomes temporarily negligible, a lapse in ego functioning which manifests itself in the clinical picture as a state of confusion.

Regression of this kind may bring transitory relief to the ego by emptying the oedipal (and many of the preoedipal) fantasies of

[5] See P. Federn (1952) and, following him, Freeman, Cameron, & McGhie (1958).

their libidinal cathexis.[6] But this lessening of anxiety will not be long-lived. Another and deeper anxiety will soon take its place which I have characterized on a former occasion (1951) as the fear of emotional surrender, with the accompanying fear of loss of identity.

(*b*) *Defence against impulses*

Where the defences against the oedipal and preoedipal object ties fail to achieve their aim, clinical pictures emerge which come nearest to the borderline towards psychotic illness.

The "ascetic" adolescent

One of these, the "ascetic" adolescent, I have described before as fighting all his impulses, preoedipal and oedipal, sexual, and aggressive, extending the defence even to the fulfilment of the physiological needs for food, sleep, and body comfort. This, to me, seems the characteristic reaction of an ego, driven by the blind fear of overwhelming id quantities, an anxiety which leaves no room for the finer distinctions between vital or merely pleasant satisfactions, the healthy or the morbid, the morally permitted or forbidden pleasures. Total war is waged against the pursuit of pleasure as such. Accordingly, most of the normal processes of instinct and need satisfaction are interfered with and become paralysed. According to clinical observation, adolescent asceticism is, with luck, a transitory phenomenon. For the analytic observer it provides precious proof of the power of defence, i.e. of the extent to which the normal, healthy drive derivatives are open to crippling interference by the ego.

On the whole, analytic treatment of the ascetic type does not present as many technical difficulties as one would expect. Perhaps, in these individuals, defence against the impulses is so massive, that they can permit themselves some object relationship to the analyst and, thus, enter into transference.

---

[6] See in this connection M. Katan (1950).

The "uncompromising" adolescent

Another equally abnormal adolescent is described best as the "uncompromising" type. The term, in this instance, does refer to more than the well-known conscious, unrelenting position adopted by many young people who stand up for their ideas, refuse to make concessions to the more practical and reality-adapted attitudes of their elders, and take pride in their moral or aesthetic principles. "Compromise", with these adolescents, includes processes which are as essential for life as, for example, the cooperation between impulses, the blending of opposite strivings, the mitigation of id strivings by interference from the side of the ego. One adolescent whom I observed in analysis did his utmost, in pursuit of this impossible aim, to prevent any interference of his mind with his body, of his activity with his passivity, his loves with his hates, his realities with his fantasies, the external demands with his internal ones, in short, of his ego with his id.

In treatment this defence was represented as a strong resistance against any "cure", the idea of which he despised in spite of intense suffering. He understood correctly that mental health is based in the last resort on harmony, i.e. on the very compromise formations which he was trying to avoid.

III. *THE CONCEPT OF NORMALITY IN ADOLESCENCE*

Where adolescence is concerned, it seems easier to describe its pathological manifestations than the normal processes. Nevertheless, there are in the above exposition at least two pronouncements which may prove useful for the concept: (1) that adolescence is by its nature an interruption of peaceful growth, and (2) that the upholding of a steady equilibrium during the adolescent process is in itself abnormal. Once we accept for adolescence disharmony within the psychic structure as our basic fact, understanding becomes easier. We begin to see the upsetting battles which are raging between id and ego as beneficent attempts to restore peace and harmony. The defensive methods which are employed either against the impulses or against the object cathexis begin to appear legitimate and normal. If they produce pathological results, this happens not because of any malignancy in their nature, but because they are overused, over-stressed, or used in isolation. Actually, each of the abnormal types of adolescent development, as it is described above, represents also a potentially useful way of regaining mental stability, normal if combined with other defences, and if used in moderation.

To explain this last statement in greater detail: I take it that it is normal for an adolescent to behave for a considerable length of time in an inconsistent and unpredictable manner; to fight his impulses and to accept them; to ward them off successfully and to be overrun by them; to love his parents and to hate them; to revolt against them and to be dependent on them; to be deeply ashamed to acknowledge his mother before others and, unexpectedly, to desire heart-to-heart talks with her; to thrive on imitation of and identification with others while searching unceasingly for his own identity; to be more idealistic, artistic, generous, and unselfish than he will ever be again, but also the opposite: self-centred, egoistic, calculating. Such fluctuations between extreme opposites would be deemed highly abnormal at any other time of life. At this time they may signify no more than that an adult structure of personality takes a long time to emerge, that the ego of the individual in question does not cease to experiment and is in no hurry to close down on possibilities. If the temporary solutions seem abnormal to the onlooker, they are less so, nevertheless, than the hasty decisions made in other cases for one-sided suppression, or revolt, or flight, or withdrawal, or regression, or asceticism, which are responsible for the truly pathological developments described above.

While an adolescent remains inconsistent and unpredictable in his behaviour, he may suffer, but he does not seem to me to be in need of treatment. I think that he should be given time and scope to work out his own solution. Rather, it may be his parents who need help and guidance so as to be able to bear with him. There are few situations in life which are more difficult to cope with than an adolescent son or daughter during the attempt to liberate themselves.

CHAPTER FOUR

On adolescence

Jeanne Lampl-de Groot

Adolescence is often regarded as a "stepchild" in psychoanalysis, in a theoretical as well as in a practical sense. A number of analysts consider the treatment of adolescent boys and girls to be very difficult, sometimes even impossible, though in some cases good results have been achieved, especially with inhibited, depressive, and compulsive–neurotic patients.

Many authors stress that our theoretical knowledge of adolescence is incomplete. I shall not review the literature in detail, but refer to the surveys of this subject by Leo Spiegel in 1951 and by Anna Freud in 1958.

Out of the many problems of adolescence, my paper will focus on two points: (1) a practical experience; and (2) some theoretical considerations, especially in connection with the formation of superego and ego ideal.

I

Anna Freud (1958) has reminded us of the fact that "our knowledge of the mental processes of infancy has been derived from reconstructions in the analyses of adults and was merely confirmed and enlarged later on by analyses or observations carried out in childhood." It is Anna Freud's opinion that in the treatment of adult cases one seldom succeeds in reviving their adolescent experiences in full force.

I think most authors will agree with this statement, and I have done so myself. However, a number of years ago two adult patients came to me for analytic treatment, a man and a woman, both in their early thirties, in whose analyses a wealth of adolescent experiences, real events as well as fantasies and impulses, came to the fore with remarkable liveliness and were accompanied by strong emotions and impulses. I hasten to add that this re-experiencing only emerged in the later phases of the analyses. In the beginning of treatment the adolescent material was brought forward merely as an account of the patient's life history in the way described by Anna Freud. The most interesting point was that the reliving of affects connected with this material did not become possible until the patient's childhood had been uncovered and reconstructed. Confronted with these observations, I recalled a statement which Freud made to me some thirty years ago. Freud told me about a young woman, who had cooperated well in her analysis and whose childhood development had been fairly well reconstructed—however, without a therapeutic result. Most of the patient's symptoms had persisted until she suddenly and vividly recollected a traumatic experience that had occurred in her fifteenth year of life. After this traumatic situation and all the emotions involved had been worked through, the patient was cured.

My own observations led me to review a number of other cases, and I gained the impression that in some of them the failure or incompleteness of success might have been due to the lack of revival of the adolescent experiences. Of course I now had to ask myself what causes might have been responsible for the fact that in these cases childhood development could be reconstructed without difficulty and re-experienced with full emotional force, whereas the adolescent period remained deprived of a full affective conviction.

From the direct study of adolescent cases we all are familiar with the charged atmosphere in which the adolescent lives, with the intensity and depth of his feelings, the sudden and unexpected mood swings, the strength of his impulses, and the force of anxiety and despair. However, are we really entitled to assume that in small children their feelings, impulses, demands, their unforeseen swings from complete happiness towards deepest sorrow and desperation are less intense than similar phenomena in adolescence?

There is indeed a difference in the demands of the instinctual drives in childhood and in adolescence, because infantile sexuality is different from genitality, which has to become the leading factor in the adolescent and adult love life.

I have the impression, however, that it is not merely the intensity of feelings, impulses, and mood swings but other factors which are more responsible for the difficulties of reviving the adolescent mental processes. These factors seem to be ego and superego development.

The little child's ego, undeveloped as it is, has to rely upon the auxiliary ego borrowed from the mother in order to master outer and inner conflicts. The superego is not yet established as an independent mental agency in infancy. Norms and restrictions are imposed upon the child by the parents. Only in the oedipal phase a structuration of the personality takes place. In latency the child develops into a more or less individual personality, though he is still dependent upon the parents. A wealth of ego capacities is established and matures during this period. In the sphere which is relatively free from conflict, intelligence, knowledge, special talents and abilities are developed, whereas in the conflictual sphere, adaptations, reaction formations, and defence mechanisms gradually become character traits. The superego as an inner institution supervises the latency child's behaviour to a large extent.

This brief outline of a child's development is very sketchy and incomplete, but it may suffice as a prelude for our considerations about adolescence.

When in puberty the instinctual drives make their new and intensified demands upon the youngster, they encounter a personality different from the one in childhood. The adolescent ego has many more ways and means of coping with the drives; in a certain sense, we could call this ego stronger. However, on the other hand, it lacks the support of the parents' auxiliary ego because the adolescent turns away from the parents. The loosening of the ties with the parents is a difficult and protracted process, often accompanied by genuine mourning, as Root (1957) and Anna Freud (1958) have pointed out. In this respect, the adolescent ego presents itself as much weaker than the child's ego. A similar process is going on with the superego. On the one hand the adolescent superego is now established as an inner conscience, on the other hand it is shaken in its foundation by the very process of turning away from the parents and the parental norms and morals. The adolescent has to rely upon his own superego. The adult, looking back upon his life history, feels more responsible for his adolescent than for his infantile behaviour; he feels more guilty and more ashamed about his adolescent conflicts, disharmonies, and oddities. As he usually remembers the factual events of adolescence, he tries to escape the revival of the accompanying guilt- and shame-burdened emotions, either by suppressing and denying every emotion of that period or by retreating to infantile experiences.

This is precisely what we often observe in analytic treatment. The patient brings us a wealth of infantile material, more and more, in different forms and associations, even when the childhood history has already been fairly well reconstructed and re-experienced. He clings tenaciously to infantile material; yet when we look at this material closely we realize that adolescent features have entered into the picture. The patient has used the infantile material in order to ward off adolescent experiences. The analyst then must analyse the defensive character of, and the underlying anxiety in regard to, this material and confront the patient with his adolescent feelings of shame, guilt, hurt pride, etc. In a number of cases the result will be a real revival of the patient's adolescence in full force.

In trying to accomplish this task we meet with difficulties, not exclusively due to the patient's reluctance to face his own adolescent problems, his unbalanced behaviour, his extreme feelings, his extravagant emotions, and his oddities. We also have to cope with the analyst's reactions to it. The analyst is prepared to meet with the patient's acting out in the transference. When the patient transfers impulses upon the analyst from his childhood period and in an infantile form, it is much easier for the latter to keep to his attitude of friendly understanding and neutrality. The adolescent has made use of all of his intelligence, capacities, and special gifts to ward off his intolerable impulses, his disappointments, and his conflicts. This is especially true in connection with his hostility towards parents, and towards adults in general. Hence, in encouraging an adult patient to relive his adolescent experiences, the analyst must cope with a refined form of the patient's aggression.

One can smile at a little child's direct form of aggressive behaviour, but an adolescent's aggression is clothed in a much more irritating, tormenting, and sometimes nearly intolerable shape. It might happen that the analyst, being a human creature himself, is (unconsciously) inclined to follow the patient in his flight towards infancy in order to escape the patient's refined criticisms, reproaches, and hostile demands. In every adult, traits not only from the little child but also from the adolescent persist. This is especially true for our patients. They tend to excuse themselves for their accusations and tormenting attacks in taking for granted that the analyst is an omnipotent and therefore invulnerable person. The interplay between the patient's anxiety to relive his adolescent emotions and conflicts and the analyst's unconscious shyness to bear the adolescent forms of aggression might be one of the causes of the difficulties we encounter in analysing and working through an adult patient's adolescence.

II

I now come to my second point: some theoretical considerations, which, I hope, will contribute to our understanding of the practical difficulties just mentioned as well as of the adolescent psychic life in general. In the scope of this presentation I can only throw light upon a few points. My assumptions are based partly on material gained in the treatment of adolescents, mainly, however, on reconstruction of adolescent experiences in adult cases.

A youngster's ego can react in an infinite variety of ways to the newly flourishing demands of his instinctual drives and to the newly arising social demands which are so different from those made upon the little child. The adolescent has on the one hand the ardent wish to be grown up because he usually imagines adults to be free, independent, and self-supporting, and he tries to use all his faculties in order to equal or even to better them. On the other hand, however, he wants to remain a little child, in order not to have to relinquish his infantile ties with the parental objects. It is very well known how difficult a task this is. Having lost a beloved person or even having renounced the love of a still existing object is followed by a certain amount of "work of mourning" [*"Trauerarbeit"*] (see Anna Freud, 1958). Whether the outcome of the mourning process will be a relatively normal or a pathological one depends upon a wealth of factors, among them upon the amount of aggression originally directed towards the parents. We know that the little child holds the parents responsible for his distress and losses, and he responds to all sorts of pain with hatred and death wishes towards his parents. When in puberty the infantile object relationships are revived, the adolescent begins to react in a similar way. The more intense his archaic hostility was, the more difficulties he will have in dealing with his death wishes. The mourning processes are coloured by the aggression turned inward. The result may be a depressive neurotic disorder, psychotic reactions, acting out or antisocial behaviour, or a combination of these various disturbances. Many authors have described several outcomes in clinical and theoretical papers.

I shall now turn to another problem of adolescence which is very different from childhood processes and nevertheless very closely dependent upon them. I mean the superego problems. I have already mentioned that in adolescence the superego has become an inner agency, whereas in early childhood behaviour was directed by the parents' demands, prohibitions, and morals. The little child cooperates with them mainly in order to avoid loss of love or punishment. Only gradually does he internalize the parental norms, which subsequently become the content of the superego. Now in adolescence he must give up his old incestuous ties to the parents—a process partly equivalent to losing the love object. But in addition he must also give up a fundamental part of his superego content—that part of the restrictions, norms, and ideals which, though internalized, are still closely linked to the incestuous object. But the very fact that these superego contents are internalized implies that the adolescent must give up something that is essentially a part of his self. To turn away from a love object is a hard and painful process; to disengage oneself from a part of one's own personality is still more difficult to achieve.

In order to examine these events more closely I propose once more to distinguish between the superego in a narrower sense as the restricting and prohibiting instance and the ego ideal as comprising norms, ethics, ideals. I have made this distinction in previous papers and it has, in my opinion, some advantages. The compliance with parental restrictions and prohibitions requires renunciation of direct pleasure, but this compliance is rewarded with love and approval from the side of the parents. The formation of ideals, however, has an additional function and has already been on the way long before parental restrictions have become internal demands. The little child idealizes the parents and conceives of them as perfect, omnipotent creatures. He clings tenaciously to these ideas because he feels himself so extremely powerless. The introjection of the almighty and faultless parental images is a compensation for the feelings of helplessness; it begins in very early childhood and is a narcissistic satisfaction par excellence. These introjected images give rise to fantasies of grandeur and omnipotence, which in the magic phase of development are among the fundamentals of the child's self-esteem and self-maintenance. It is well known that part of the feelings of grandeur continue to exist, though unconsciously, throughout life.

The adolescent must bear not only the pain of losing love objects, of coping with the attending mourning, and of revising old patterns of restriction and prohibition. In addition to all these hard tasks, he must endure the narcissistic injuries caused by his self-esteem being shaken in its fundamentals and therefore more or less lost. We know too well that a certain amount of narcissistic cathexis of the personality is indispensable for a healthy development. When the basis of the ideal formation has gone to pieces, the youngster is utterly helpless. I hasten to add that the loss of love is of course partly felt as a narcissistic injury as well. The finding of a new love object raises the person's self-esteem, too. However, it seems to make a considerable difference when an essential part of the ego (ego ideal) is damaged or lost and has to be newly built up. New love objects are relatively easily found in adolescence in teachers, leaders, companions, etc. New ideals that compensate for the essential helplessness of human beings are more difficult to acquire (at least in our civilization). The youngster very well knows, and feels, that adults are not omnipotent but vulnerable creatures. We find a confirmation of this assumption in studying those adolescents who do not respond to offers of love and guidance from a new object (relative, teacher, therapist, companion, etc.). These youngsters could not overcome the depth of their inner narcissistic injuries; consequently they are indifferent to supplies of love from the outer world. It is possible that a number of strange reactions, of unexpected attitudes and unpredictable mood swings are due to this basic disturbance in the economy of narcissistic libido and the ego's failure to restore it. Moreover, it is just the narcissistic injuries that are pre-eminently apt to give rise to aggression, and this hostility in its turn diminishes a person's susceptibility to another person's loving assistance or the offer of new ideals and norms.

In the transference during treatment we can observe that a patient's deep and refined hostility, severe criticisms of the analyst, reproaches that the analyst is impotent and worthless go side by side with an unconscious, archaic conviction of the analyst's omnipotence. The ideal image of almighty parents and analysts not only is indispensable for the youngster's maintenance of narcissistic cathexis, but it is secondarily used in order to diminish the guilt feelings aroused by precisely this same hostile and aggressive behaviour. It is as if the youngster says to himself: "Parents and analyst are omnipotent, consequently they are invulnerable; so I can scold, torment, and act out every aggression without having to feel guilty or reproach myself."

It would be tempting to illustrate these assumptions with detailed analytic material. However, in this paper, I merely wanted to emphasize the importance of the problems around the ego ideal in adolescence. The adolescent's clinging to the very archaic, idealized parental images makes it so difficult for him to cope with the narcissistic injuries occasioned by the necessity of having to give them up and finding new ideals in a more reality-adapted form. Furthermore, he needs to hold on to this idealized picture because it also serves as a defence against guilt and shame engendered by the intense hostility.

When many analysts agree that adolescent patients are often not suitable for analytic treatment, we must, in our attempts to understand adolescent psychology, rely mainly on observations and reconstructions of adolescence in adult cases. But even these reconstructions, as has been pointed out, are extremely difficult to achieve. This paper has endeavoured to investigate some of the obstacles in the way of such reconstruction and to indicate means of overcoming them.

I believe that we might be successful in reviving adolescence in a number of cases if we make an effort to overcome our own resistance against the patient's adolescent forms of aggression, if we focus our and the patient's attention upon his hidden ideals and fantasies of omnipotence attributed to his parents and later on internalized, and if we support the patient in enduring his narcissistic hurts and in giving up the defensive character of his archaic ideal. I believe that this effort is worth while.

CHAPTER FIVE

The second individuation process of adolescence

Peter Blos

The biological processes of growth and differentiation during puberty effect changes in the structure and in the functioning of the organism. These changes occur in a typical and sequential order, called maturation. The same applies to the psychological changes of adolescence. These, too, follow a developmental pattern but of a different order, since these changes draw content, stimulation, aim, and direction from a complex interplay of inner and outer impingements. What we, eventually, observe are new stabilizing processes and alterations of psychic structures, both of which are the result of adolescent accommodations.

At the points where both the pubertal maturation and the adolescent accommodation intersect in order to become integrated, there we find the critical stations of adolescent development. I have described these stations, clinically and theoretically, in terms of adolescent phases (Blos, 1962). They are the milestones of progressive development, each marked by a phase-specific conflict, a maturational task, and a resolution that is preconditional for the advance to higher levels of differentiation. Beyond these typical aspects of the adolescent phases, we can recognize a component in psychic restructuring that winds, like a scarlet thread, through the entire fabric of adolescence. This unrelenting component is manifest with equal pertinacity in preadolescence as in late adolescence. It is conceptualized here as the second individuation process of adolescence. In my previous studies of adolescence I have continuously emphasized the heterogeneity of phases in terms of the positions and movements of drive and ego. My attention turns now to a process of a more pervasive order whose sameness in direction and in aim extends without letup through the entire period of adolescence.

I propose to view adolescence in its totality as the second individuation process, the first one having been completed towards the end of the third year of life with the attainment of object constancy. Both periods have in common a heightened vulnerability of the personality organization. Both periods have in common the urgency for changes in psychic structure in consonance with the maturational forward surge. Last but not least, both periods—should they miscarry—are followed by a specific deviant development (psychopathology) that embodies the respective failures of individuation. What is in infancy a "hatching from the symbiotic membrane to become an individuated toddler" (Mahler, 1963) becomes in adolescence the shedding of family dependencies, the loosening of infantile object ties in order to become a member of society at large or, simply, of the adult world. In metapsychological terms, we would say that not until the termination of adolescence do self and object representations acquire stability and firm boundaries, i.e. they become resistant to cathectic shifts. The oedipal superego—in contrast to the archaic superego—loses in the process some of its rigidity and power, while the narcissistic institution of the ego ideal acquires more pervasive prominence and influence. The maintenance of the narcissistic balance is thus further internalized. These structural changes establish constancy of self-esteem and of mood as increasingly independent from external sources or, at best, dependent on the external sources of one's own choosing.

The disengagement from internalized objects—love and hate objects—opens the way in adolescence to the finding of external and extrafamilial love and hate objects. The reverse was true in early childhood during the separation–individuation phase, when the child gained psychological separateness from a concrete object, the mother. This was achieved through the process of internalization that gradually facilitated the child's growing independence from the mother's presence, her ministrations, and her emotional supplies as the chief and sole regulators of psychophysiological homeostasis. The progress from the symbiotic oneness of child and mother to that of separateness from her is marked by the formation of internal regulatory capacities which are assisted and promoted by maturational—especially motor, perceptual, verbal, and cognitive—advances. This process is at best a pendular one, as we observe again in the second individuation process of adolescence. Regressive and progressive movements alternate in shorter or longer intervals, easily giving the casual observer of the child a lopsided maturational impression. Only observation over a period of time enables us to judge the behaviour of the average toddler or of the average adolescent as to its normal or deviant nature.

Adolescent individuation is the reflection of those structural changes that accompany the emotional disengagement from internalized infantile objects. The complexity of this process has been, for some time, in the centre of analytic attention. In fact, it is by now axiomatic that without a successful disengagement from infantile internalized objects, the finding of new, namely extra-familial, love objects in the outside world is either precluded, hindered, or remains restricted to simple replication and substitution. The ego is intrinsically involved in this process because, up to adolescence, the parental ego is selectively available to the child and, indeed, is his legitimate ego extension. This condition is an integral aspect of childhood dependency in the service of anxiety control and self-esteem regulation. With the disengagement from infantile libidinal dependencies in adolescence, the accustomed ego dependencies of the latency period are repudiated as well. Therefore, the ego weakness of adolescence is not only due to the increasing strength of the drives but, in large measure, to the disengagement from the parental ego support. Up to adolescence this support constitutes an essential component of the child's ego. Relative ego weakness due to the intensification of the drives, as well as absolute ego weakness due to the reduction of parental ego support are both enmeshed in our clinical observations. The recognition of these disparate elements of adolescent ego weakness is of theoretical interest but also of practical usefulness in our analytic work. A case illustration will clarify this point.

A young adolescent boy, tormented by castration anxiety, had borrowed his mother's magical defence that says: "Nothing bad will ever happen as long as you don't think about it." The boy's use of thought control in the service of anxiety management revealed two components, inextricably linked together. The drive component resided in the boy's masochistic submission to his mother's will and advice, while his ego had borrowed the mother's magic in order to free itself from intense anxiety. The child's ego had identified with the mother's anxiety-control system. With the advent of puberty the renewed and, indeed, frantic employment of the mother's magic only increased his dependency on her, thus indicating the only course his sexual drive could take, namely, infantile, sadomasochistic dependency. In freeing himself from the dependency on his mother by using her magic device, he made himself the victim of her omnipotence by sharing her falsification of reality. The libidinization of submission obstructed progressive development. The magic device could become ego alien only after the ego had gained in critical self-observation and in reality testing. To say it differently: only after the castration anxiety in relation to the archaic mother was recognized could the phallic modality assert itself and counteract the passive submissive trend. On the ego level, this shift in drive orientation appeared as a repudiation of the magical fallacy whose prototype was the omnipotent mother of infancy. A growing capacity of reality testing went parallel with the repudiation of infantile ego positions, thus enlarging the scope of the autonomous ego.

The disengagement from the infantile object is always paralleled by ego maturation. The reverse is equally true, namely, that adolescent inadequacy or impairment of ego functions is symptomatic of drive fixations and infantile object dependencies. The accumulative ego alterations that parallel drive progression in each adolescent phase accrue in a structural innovation that is identified here as the second individuation.

Without doubt, there appear during adolescence unique and new ego capacities or faculties, such as, for instance, the spectacular advances in the cognitive sphere (Inhelder & Piaget, 1958). However, observation has left us wondering as to their nature of primary autonomy and, furthermore, as to their independence from drive maturation. Experience teaches us that, whenever drive development lags critically behind adolescent ego differentiation, the newly acquired ego functions are, without fail, drawn into defensive employment and lose their autonomous character. Conversely, an advance in drive maturation affects ego differentiation and functioning favourably. The interacting stimulation between drive and ego proceeds most vigorously and effectively if both operate and progress within an optional proximity of each other. Both drive and ego development exert a continuous influence on each other. The loosening of the infantile object ties not only makes way for more mature or age-adequate relationships, but simultaneously the ego in turn becomes increasingly antagonistic to the re-establishment of outmoded and partly abandoned ego states and drive gratifications of childhood.

Analysts familiar with adolescents have always been impressed by the central concern which relationships occupy in the life of the adolescent. The intensity and extent of object-directed drive manifestations or the intensity and extent of object-directed drive inhibition should, however, not obscure the radical alterations in ego structure that take place during this time. The sum total of these structural changes survives adolescence as enduring personality attributes.

What I endeavour to convey is the particular character of psychic restructuring in adolescence when shifts in object libido bring about ego alterations, which in turn give the process of object losing and object finding ("pushing away" and "holding on") not only a greater urgency but also a broader adaptive scope. This circular response has normally diminished by the close of adolescence with the result that the ego has acquired its distinct and definitive organization. Within this organization there remains a wide scope open for elaborations during adult life. The ego ideal affects these elaborations decisively.

We are now eager to trace the steps of individuation during adolescence. In studying this process we have learned much from those adolescents who side-step the transformation of psychic structure and replace the disengagement from internal objects by a polarization to them in the form of idiosyncratic behaviour and social role. Ego disturbances, apparent in acting out, in learning disorders, in lack of purpose, in procrastination, in moodiness and negativism, are frequently the symptomatic signs of a failure in the disengagement from infantile objects, and, consequently, they represent a failure of individuation itself. As clinicians we recognize in the adolescent's wholesale rejection of his family and of his own past the frantic circumvention of the painful disengagement process. Such avoidances are usually transient, and the delays are self-liquidating. They might, however, assume extreme forms. We are familiar with the adolescent who runs away, drives off in a stolen car, leaves school, "bums" his way to nowhere, takes to promiscuity and to drugs. These adolescents have usually removed themselves, emphatically and with finality, from their families, convinced that no useful communication is possible between the generations. In the assessment of such cases one often arrives at the conclusion that the adolescent is "doing the wrong thing for the right reasons". One cannot fail but recognize in the emergency measures of a violent rupture with childhood and family continuities the escape from an overwhelming regressive pull to infantile dependencies, grandiosities, safeties, and gratifications. The effort to separate from infantile dependencies is in consonance with the adolescent task: the means employed, however, are bound to abort the maturational momentum.

For many adolescents this violent rupture constitutes a respite, a holding position, until progressive development is rekindled again. For many, however, it becomes a way of life which sooner or later leads back to what, at the outset, was to be avoided, namely, regression. By forcing a physical, geographic, moral, and ideational distance from the family or the locale of childhood, this type of adolescent renders an internal separation dispensable. In his actual separateness and independence he experiences an intoxicating sense of triumph over his past and slowly becomes addicted to his state of apparent liberation. The countercathectic energy employed in upholding this state of life accounts for the often striking inefficacy, emotional shallowness, procrastination, and expectant suspense which characterize the various forms of individuation avoidance. True enough, the physical separateness from the parent or the polarization with the past through change in social role, style of dress and grooming, special interests, and moral choices often represent the only means by which the adolescent can maintain his psychological integrity during some critical stages of the individuation process. The degree of maturity ultimately attained depends on how far the individuation process advanced or where it came to an impasse and was left incomplete. It follows from the above that the second individuation is a relative concept: on the one hand, it depends on drive maturation and, on the other hand, it acquires durability in ego structure. The second individuation, therefore, connotes those ego changes that are the accompaniment and the consequence of the adolescent disengagement from infantile objects.

Individuation implies that the growing person takes increasing responsibility for what he does and what he is, rather than depositing this responsibility onto the shoulders of those under whose influence and tutelage he has grown up. In our times it has become a pervasive attitude of the more sophisticated adolescent to blame the parent for the shortcomings and disappointments of his youth or, on a transcendental scale, to see in the uncontrollable powers of various designations the ultimate and absolute forces that govern life. It appears senseless to the adolescent who has taken such a position to rise against these forces, but he rather declares a resigned purposelessness of such an effort the true hallmark of maturity. It is the Camusian stance of the protagonist in *The Stranger*. The incapacity to separate from internal objects except by detachment, rejection, and debasement is subjectively experienced as a sense of alienation. We recognize in it the endemic mood of a considerable segment of present-day adolescents, promising and gifted sons and daughters, having grown up in ambitious, yet indulgent, usually middle-class, often progressive and liberal families. In studying the morphology of adolescent individuation in historical perspective we come to realize that each epoch evolves predominant roles and styles through which this adolescent task is implemented and socialized. Such epiphenomena of the individuation process always stand in opposition to the established order, in one way or another.[1] It remains a crucial difference whether this new way of life becomes the displaced battleground of liberation from childhood dependencies, thus leading to individuation, or whether the new forms become permanent substitutions of childhood states, thus precluding progressive development. The pathognomic valence of a physical separation like "running away", "leaving school", or rushing into all sorts of adultomorphic, especially sexual, forms of life can be determined only if viewed in relation to the individual life history, to the total milieu and its traditional sanctions of the behavioural forms that give expression to pubertal needs. Pubertal drive intensification reactivates primary object relations within the context of certain preferential, pregenital drive modalities. However, libido and aggression do not simply shift in an about-face move from primary love objects to non-incestuous ones during adolescence. All along, the ego is intrinsically involved in these cathectic shifts, and it acquires in the process the structure by which the post-adolescent personality is defined. Adolescent individuation, then, reflects a process and an achievement, both of which constitute integral components of the total adolescent process.

I shall now leave the description of familiar adolescent accommodations and turn to a discussion of their theoretical implications. The process of disengagement from infantile objects, so essential for progressive development, renews the ego's contact with infantile drive and infantile ego positions. The post-latency ego is, so to say, prepared for this regressive encounter and capable

[1]As example, one might think of the ostentatiously simple and comfortable clothes introduced by a faction of educated German male youth during the second half of the eighteenth century as a reaction to the French refinement and daintiness of men's clothing. Tearing off the delicate laces from their shirt-fronts was complemented by an affectation of exuberant emotionality between male youths (tears, embraces) and a replacement of the wig by free-flowing natural hair. The influence of Rousseau as well as a reaction to the "Phoniness of the Establishment" is traceable in that segment of youth that created its own unconventional and natural style and, beyond that, furnished its part to the political ferment of the times.

of different, more stable and age-adequate solutions of infantile predilections. The reinstatement of infantile positions, ego and drive positions, is an essential component of the adolescent disengagement process. Relatively stable ego functions, for example, memory or motor control, and, furthermore, relatively stable psychic institutions, for example, the superego, will undergo remarkable fluctuations and changes in their executive functions. The trained observer can recognize in the transient breakdown and in the final reconstitution of these functions and institutions their ontogenetic history. One is tempted to speak, mechanistically, of an adolescent reassemblage of the psychic components within the framework of a fixed psychic apparatus. The superego, once considered an inflexible post-oedipal institution, undergoes considerable reorganization during adolescence (A. Freud, 1952). The analytic observation of superego changes has been most instructive for studying the mutability of psychic structure. We shall now look closer at the changeability of this post-oedipal institution. The regressive personification of the superego appears in great clarity during the analysis of adolescents. This permits us to glance at its origin in object relations. The unravelling of the process that led to superego formation is like a film played backward. Excerpts from the analysis of two adolescents will illustrate this. Both of them were unable to conform with any routine requirements of daily life; both of them were failures in work of any kind, and, also, in love of any kind.

1. An older adolescent boy became puzzled by the fact that he is equally neglectful of what he likes to do as of what he dislikes to do. The latter he could easily understand, but the former made no sense to him. He became aware of a preconscious thought that accompanied his activity or the choice of it. He asked himself: "Would my mother consider what I do a good thing; would she want me to do it?" The affirmative thought automatically spoiled the activity, even if it was one of a pleasurable nature. At this impasse he became totally inactive. He continued the recounting of this dilemma by saying: "When I know that my mother wants me to do what I want to do—namely, if we both want the same—then I get embarrassed and I stop whatever I am doing."

2. An older adolescent girl, who all through childhood had guided her actions to win the praise and admiration of those close to her, embarked in her late adolescence on a way of life that stood in stark opposition to family standards and style. She had stopped to be what she thought others wanted her to be. To her distress, her self-chosen independence afforded her no sense of self-determination because, at every turn, the thought of her parents' approval or disapproval intervened. Her decisions, so she felt, were not her own, because they were guided by doing the obverse of what would please her parents. A total stalemate of action and decision making was the result. She drifted hither and yon in the fickle breeze of circumstances. All she could do was to delegate parental guidance to her friends of both sexes, living vicariously by their expectancies and gratifications, while being tormented by the constant fear of succumbing to their influence or, on a deeper level, of merging and losing her sense of self.

In both cases the enmeshment of the superego with infantile object relations resulted in a developmental impasse. What, normally, is accomplished during latency, namely, the reduction of infantile object dependency through identification and through the organization of the superego, had failed to succeed in both cases I have mentioned. Instead, primitive identifications, as those laid down in the archaic superego and in precursory stages of the superego, had left their powerful imprint on these two adolescents. Uniqueness fantasies and grandiose self-expectations, once realized through identification with the omnipotent mother, made all goal-directed action painfully insignificant and disappointing. The adolescent task of superego reorganization threw these two adolescents back onto the archaic level of primitive identifications (Reich, 1954). The origin of the superego in oedipal and in preoedipal object relations renders this institution the subject for a radical revision in adolescence. It is no wonder that superego disturbances constitute a uniquely adolescent deviancy. Whenever the secondary autonomy of ego functions has only tenuously been achieved in childhood, object libido continues to gain gratification in their exercise. This heritage will throw superego functions into a disastrous disarray with the advance of pubertal maturation. Should adolescent behaviour be dictated, massively and lastingly, by a defence against infantile object gratification, then the adolescent reorganization of the superego is precluded or, in other words, adolescent individuation remains incomplete.

Analytic work with adolescents demonstrates, almost monotonously, the reinvolvement of ego and superego functions with infantile object relations. The study of this subject has convinced me that the danger to ego integrity does not derive alone from the strength of the pubertal drives, but comes, in equal measure, from the strength of the regressive pull. Discounting the assumption of a fundamental enmity between ego and id, I came to the conclusion that the task of psychic restructuring by regression represents the most formidable psychic work of adolescence. Just as Hamlet longs for the comforts of sleep but fears the dreams that sleep might bring, so the adolescent longs for the comforts of drive gratification but fears the reinvolvements in infantile object relations. Paradoxically, only through regression and drive and ego regression can the adolescent task be fulfilled. This is made feasible through the ego differentiation or ego maturation that is the normal heritage of the latency period. The reality-bound and self-observing part of the ego is normally kept, at least marginally, intact during the regressive movements of adolescence. Thus the dangers of regression are reduced or regulated, averting the catastrophic danger of the regressive loss of self, of a return to the undifferentiated stage, or of merger. However, only through regression at adolescence can the residues of infantile trauma, conflict, or fixation be modified by bringing to bear on them the ego's extended resources that draw, at this age, support from the developmental momentum of growth and maturation.

Geleerd (1961) has suggested that "in adolescence a partial regression to the undifferentiated phase of object relationship occurs". In a later paper, based on this earlier study, Geleerd (1964) has broadened her view and stated that "the growing individual passes through many regressive stages in which all three structures participate". This last-mentioned formulation has been affirmed by clinical work and is by now an integral part of the psychoanalytic theory of adolescence. Hartmann (1939) had laid the foundation for these developmental considerations in his formulation of "regressive adaptation". This adaptive modality plays a role throughout life in all kinds of situations.

What I emphasize here is the fact that adolescence is the only period in human life during which ego regression and drive regression constitute an obligatory component of normal development. Adolescent regression operates, therefore, in the service of development. Furthermore, the subject of my investigation is the mutual influence of, or the interaction between, ego and drive regression as they effect changes in psychic structure. The process and the achievement of those structural changes are conceptualized here as adolescent individuation, emphasizing the prominent role of the decathexis of infantile object representations in adolescent psychic restructuring. The phase-specific regression initiates transient, maladaptive hazards and maintains a state of high psychic volatility in youth (Blos, 1963). This condition accounts for much of the perplexing behaviour and the unique emotional turbulence of this age.

In order to expound further the function of adolescent regression it might be useful to compare it with the regressive movements of early childhood. States of stress that overtax the child's adaptive capacity are in early childhood normally responded to by drive and ego regression. Regressions of this nature do not, however, constitute developmental steps that are preconditional to ego and drive maturation. In contrast, adolescent regression, which is not defensive in nature, constitutes an integral part of development at puberty. This regression, nevertheless, induces anxiety more often than not. Should this anxiety become unmanageable, then, secondarily, defensive measures become mobilized. Regression in adolescence is not, in and by itself, a defence, but it constitutes an essential psychic process that, despite the anxiety it engenders, must take its course. Only then can the task be fulfilled that is implicit in adolescent development. It cannot be emphasized enough that what, initially, in this process serves a defensive or restitutive function turns, normally, into an adaptive one and contributes decisively to the uniqueness of a given personality.

In the process of psychic restructuring we observe not only drive regression but also ego regression as a universal by-play of the adolescent individuation process. Ego regression connotes the re-experiencing of abandoned or partly abandoned ego states which had been either citadels of safety and security, or which once had constituted special ways of coping with stress. Ego regression is always in evidence in the adolescent process, but only as far as it operates purely defensively does it work against the evolvement of individuation. We cannot but recognize, retrospectively, in many an adolescent's vagary, that a strategic retreat was the surest road to victory. *Reculer pour mieux sauter*. Only when drive and ego regression reach the immobility of an adolescent fixation does progressive development come to a standstill.

Ego regression is, for example, to be found in the re-experiencing of traumatic states of which no childhood was ever wanting. In self-contrived confrontations with miniature editions or proxy representations of the original trauma in real life situations, the ego gradually acquires mastery over prototypical danger situations. Adolescent play-acting and experimentation as well as much of delinquent pathology belong to this, often maladaptive, ego activity. Normally, a broadened ego autonomy ensues from the struggle against and with the remnants of childhood trauma. From this point of view, adolescence can be contemplated as offering a second chance for coming to terms with overwhelming danger situations (in relation to id, superego, and reality) that have survived the periods of infancy and childhood.

Adolescent ego states of a regressed nature can be recognized in a return to "action language" as distinguished from verbal, i.e. symbolic communication and, furthermore, in a return to "body language", to somatization of affects, conflicts, and drives. This latter condition is responsible for the many typical physical complaints and conditions of adolescence, which are epitomized in anorexia nervosa and in psychogenic obesity. This is particularly evident in girls, in contrast to boys; it is part of that libidinal diffusion that effects in the female the erotization of the body, especially its surface. Object libido deflected on body parts or organ systems facilitates the formation of "hypochondriacal sensations and feelings of body changes that are well known clinically from initial stages of psychotic illness" (A. Freud, 1958).

Contemplating the "action language" of adolescent behaviour, one cannot fail but recognize in it the problem of active versus passive. This antithesis constitutes the earliest one in individual life. It is not surprising that with the onset of puberty, with the bewildering crescendo of instinctual tension, the adolescent falls back on old and familiar modes of tension reduction. Drive regression, in search of one of these modes, leads ultimately to primal passivity. This stands in fatal opposition to the maturing body, to its emerging physical competencies as well as to newly unfolding mental capabilities. Progressive development points to an increasing degree of self-reliance, to an ever greater mastery of the environment, indeed, to its transformation, thus bringing the realization of desires and aspirations within reach.

Regressed ego states are identifiable also in the well-known adolescent idolization and adoration of famous men and women. In our contemporary world they are, predominantly, chosen from show business and sports. These figures are the collective great ones. We are reminded of the idealized parent of the child's younger years. Their glorified images constituted an indispensable regulator of the child's narcissistic balance. It should not surprise us that the bedroom walls, plastered with the collective idols, become bare as soon as object libido is engaged in genuine relationships. Then, the pictorial flock of transient gods and goddesses is rendered dispensable almost overnight.

Infantile ego states are, furthermore, recognizable in the emotional state that is akin to merger. Such states are frequently experienced, e.g. in relation to abstractions such as Truth, Nature, Beauty, or in the involvement with ideas or ideals of a political, philosophical, aesthetic, or religious nature. Such ego states of quasi-merger in the realm of symbolic representations are sought as temporary respite and serve as safeguards against total merger with the infantile internalized objects. Religious conversions or merger states induced by drugs belong to this realm of ego regression.

Ego regression to the stage where self and inner object merge is a pathognomic phenomenon because, normally, the ego component to which we refer as the critical and observing ego continues to exercise its function, even if conspicuously diminished, and thus prevents ego regression from deteriorating into an infantile state of merger. Limited ego regression, typical as well as obligatory in adolescence, can occur only within a relatively intact ego. There is no doubt that adolescent ego regression puts the ego to a severe test. It has been pointed out earlier that, up to adolescence, the parental ego makes itself available to the child and lends structure and organization to its ego as a functional entity. Adolescence disrupts this alliance, and ego regression lays bare the intactness or defectiveness of the early ego organization, which derived decisive positive and negative qualities from the passage through the first separation–individuation phase in the second and third year of life. Adolescent ego regression within a defective ego structure engulfs the regressed ego in its early abnormal condition. The distinction between the pathognomic and normal nature of ego regression lies precisely in the alternative whether ego regression to the undifferentiated stage is approximated or consummated. This distinction is comparable to that between a dream and a hallucination. The regression to a seriously defective ego of early childhood will turn a developmental impasse, so typical of adolescence, into a temporary or permanent psychotic illness. The degree of early ego inadequacy often does not become apparent until adolescence, when regression fails to serve progressive development, precludes individuation, and closes the door to drive and ego maturation.

In following the development of schizophrenic children whom I had treated successfully in early and middle childhood, I became aware of the fact that they encountered a more or less serious recurrence of their early pathology in late adolescence. This usually occurred at the time of their leaving home after they had made in the intervening years remarkable strides in their psychological development. The developmental function of adolescent ego regression came to naught when early ego states, from which the second individuation process must draw its strength, were reactivated in these children. The nuclear pathology flared up once more. The failure of the emotional disengagement from the family during adolescence demonstrated how extensively these children had lived on borrowed ego strength in the intervening years. Therapy had enabled them to derive emotional nurture from the environment. This capacity stood them in good stead during their second acute illness; indeed, it carried them through and made their recovery possible. When the psychological navel cord has to be cut in adolescence, children with early ego damage fall back on a defective psychic structure that is totally inadequate to the task of the adolescent individuation process. While these cases throw light on the structural problems of a certain adolescent psychopathology, they also hint at a treatment continuum of childhood psychosis or childhood schizophrenia, reaching into or having to be resumed again in the adolescent, usually the late adolescent years.

A characteristic of adolescence that cannot escape our notice lies in a frantic effort to keep reality-bound, i.e. to be active, to move about, and to keep doing things. Furthermore, it appears in the need for group experiences or individual relationships of vivid and acute excitement and affectivity. The frequent and often abrupt change of these relationships with either sex highlights their ungenuine character. What is sought is not the personal bond but the sharpness of affect and the emotional agitation evoked by it. Into this realm belongs the pressing need to do things "for kicks", thus escaping affective loneliness, dullness, and boredom. This picture would be incomplete without mentioning the adolescent who seeks solitude and splendid isolation where he conjures up in his mind affective states of extraordinary intensity. These propensities are best designated as affect and object hunger. What all these adolescents have in common is the need for sharp, intense affective states, be they marked by exuberance and elation or pain and anguish. We can look at this affective condition as a restitutive phenomenon that follows in the wake of internal object loss and the concomitant ego impoverishment.[2] The subjective experience of the adolescent, expressed in the quandary of "Who am I?" contains multitudinous perplexities and reflects what is conceptualized as ego loss and ego impoverishment. Ego loss, then, remains throughout adolescence a constant threat to psychological integrity and gives rise to forms of behaviour that appear deviant but need to be assessed as efforts to keep the adolescent process in motion by a frantic—event if maladaptive—turn to reality. The

[2] It seems, at first sight, a contradiction to speak of "ego impoverishment" when object libido is deflected on the self. However, a healthy ego cannot tolerate well and for long being cut off from object relations. The flooding of the self with narcissistic libido becomes ego syntonic only in the psychotic adolescent; for him, the real world is dull and colourless. The "normal" adolescent experiences a sense of frightening unreality in mounting narcissistic isolation from the object world. Masturbation, therefore, can never offer a permanent form of gratification because, eventually, it lowers self-esteem.

clinical picture of many a delinquent, if viewed within this perspective, reveals often more of a healthy component than he is usually credited with.

I shall, once more, consider adolescent object hunger and ego impoverishment. Both these developmental transient conditions find compensatory relief in the group, the gang, the coterie, the contemporaries generally. This social formation is a substitute, often literally, of the adolescent's family. Within the society of the contemporaries lies stimulation, belongingness, loyalty, devotion, empathy, and resonance. I am here reminded of the healthy toddler in Mahler's study (1963) who shows during the separation–individuation crisis an amazing capacity to "extract contact supplies and participation from the mother". This contact supply in adolescence is obtained from the group of contemporaries. The toddler requires the help of the mother to reach autonomy, while the adolescent turns to the contemporary horde, of whatever type it may be, to extract those contact supplies without which individuation cannot be realized. The group permits identifications as role tryouts without any permanent commitment, as well as interactional experimentation as severance actions from childhood dependencies, rather than as preludes to any new and permanent, personal and intimate relationship. Furthermore, the group shares and thus alleviates individual guilt feelings that accompany the emancipation from childhood dependencies, prohibitions, and loyalties. We can summarize and say that, by and large, the contemporaries ease the way to membership in the new generation within which the adolescent has to establish his social, personal, and sexual identity. Whenever peer relationships simply replace childhood dependencies, then the group has miscarried its function. In such cases, the adolescent process has been short-circuited, with the result that unresolved emotional dependencies are made permanent personality attributes. Under these circumstances life within the new generation unfolds strangely like a shadow play of the individual past: what was to be avoided most repeats itself with fateful accuracy.

An older adolescent girl, stalemated in a massive anti-conformity position that served as a protection against an unusually strong regressive pull, put so well into words what I have endeavoured to convey that I shall let her speak. In contemplating an instance of nonconformity, she said: "If you act in opposition to what is expected, you bump right and left into regulations and rules. Today, when I ignored school—just didn't go—it made me feel very good. It gave me a sense of being a person, not just an automaton. If you continue to rebel and bump into the world around you often enough, then an outline of yourself gets drawn in your mind. You need that. Maybe, when you know who you are, you don't have to be different from those who know, or think they know, who you should be."

I shall now turn to the broader consequences of the fact that regression in adolescence is the precondition for progressive development. I inferred from clinical observations that the adolescent has to come into emotional contact with the passions of his infancy and early childhood in order for them to surrender their original cathexes; only then can the past fade into conscious and unconscious memories, and only then will the forward movement of the libido give youth that unique emotional intensity and power of purpose.

The profoundest and most unique quality of adolescence lies in its capacity to move between regressive and progressive consciousness with an ease that has no equal at any other period in human life. This might account for the remarkable creative achievements of this particular age. The adolescent experimentation with self and reality, with feeling states and thoughts will accrue, if all goes well, in giving a lasting and precise content and form to individuation in terms of its actualization on the environment. The choice of a vocation, for example, represents one such crucial form of actualization.

In the process of disengagement from primary love and hate objects, a quality of early object relations appears in the form of ambivalence. The clinical picture of adolescence demonstrates the defusion of instinctual drives. Acts of raw aggression are typical of adolescence in general and of male adolescence in particular. The analysis of these aggressive manifestations leads ultimately to elements of infantile rage and sadism—in essence, to infantile ambivalence. Infantile object relations, when revived at adolescence, are bound to appear in their original form, which is to say, in an ambivalent state. Indeed, it remains the ultimate task of adolescence to strengthen post-ambivalent object relations. The emotional instability of relationships and, above and beyond that, the inundation of autonomous ego functions by ambivalence generally creates in the adolescent a state of precarious lability and incomprehensible contradictions in affect, drive, thought, and behaviour. The emotional fluctuations between the extremes of love and hate, of activity and passivity, of fascination and lack of interest represent a characteristic of adolescence so well known that it requires no elaboration. However, this phenomenon is worth exploring in relation to the subject of this investigation, namely, individuation. A state of ambivalence confronts the ego with a condition that—due to the ego's relatively mature state—is felt as intolerable, yet it remains, temporarily at least, beyond the ego's synthesizing capacity to deal with this condition constructively. Much that appears to be a defensive operation, such as negativism, oppositionalism, indifference, etc., is but a manifestation of an ambivalent state that has pervaded the total personality.

Before pursuing these thoughts any further, I shall illustrate them with an excerpt from the analysis of a seventeen-year-old boy. I shall concentrate in what follows on those aspects of the analytic material that reflect the disengagement from the archaic mother and that have a direct bearing on the topic of ambivalence and individuation. The boy, able and intelligent, related on an intellectualizing level to people—better to adults than to peers. A passive–aggressive attitude pervaded his contact with people, especially within the family. One became aware of a tumultuous inner life that had found no expression in affective behaviour. The boy was given to moodiness, secretiveness, uneven work performance in school, periodic stubbornness, and negativism, coupled with a cold demandingness at home. Within this fluctuating picture one could discern an all-pervasive haughty, impenetrable superciliousness that bordered on arrogance. This abnormal state was well fortified by compulsive-obsessional defences. The choice of this defence in and by itself hints at the dominant role of ambivalence in the pathogenesis of this case.

Not until the boy's fantasies became accessible was it possible to appreciate his need for a rigid and unassailable defence organization. His every act and thought was accompanied by a—heretofore unconscious—involvement with the mother and her fantasied complicity, good or bad, in his daily life. He had possessed an insatiable need for closeness to his mother, who had left him from early life on in the care of a well-meaning relative. The boy had always admired, envied, and praised his mother. The analysis helped him experience his hate, contempt, and fear in relation to her whenever his intense wishes for her material generosity were thwarted. It became clear that his actions and moods were determined by the ebb and flow of love and hate that he felt towards his mother or that he imagined his mother felt towards him. In consequence, for example, he would not do his homework when the thought prevailed that his academic achievement would please his mother. At other times it was the reverse. When he received a reward at school, he kept it a secret from his mother, so she could not use his achievement as a "feather in her own cap" or, in other words, take it away from him. When he went for a walk, he did so in secret, because his mother preferred an outdoor boy and, to put her in the wrong, he would then let her scold him for not getting any fresh air. Should he enjoy a show or invite a friend, it ruined the pleasure of the event when the mother showed delight and approval. In retaliation, he practised the piano, as he was supposed to do, but played the pieces fortissimo, knowing well that the loud sound would get on his mother's nerves. Playing loudly substituted for shouting at her. The realization of his aggression made him anxious.

At this point, the analysis of the boy's ambivalence became blocked by a narcissistic defence. He experienced himself as being an outsider to the drama of life, of being uninvolved in the events of the day, and of seeing his surroundings in blurred and fuzzy outlines. The usual compulsive-obsessional defences (like cataloguing, filing, repairing) failed in coping with this emergency. He found this state of depersonalization quite unpleasant and disconcerting. The analytic work began to flow again when he became aware of the sadistic aspect of his ambivalence. Then, the strange ego state left him. He felt and verbalized his impulse towards violence, namely, to strike out and hurt his mother physically whenever she frustrated him. The sense of frustration was not dependent on her objective actions but rather on the ebb and flow of his needs. The replication of infantile ambivalence was apparent. He was now able to differentiate between the mother of the infantile period and the mother of the present situation. This enabled us to trace the involvement of ego functions in his adolescent ambivalence conflict and bring about the restoration of their autonomy.

It was interesting to observe how in the resolution of the ambivalence conflict certain selected attributes of the mother's personality became attributes of the boy's ego, such as her capacity to work, her use of intelligence, and her able sociability, which all had been the objects of the son's envy. On the other hand, some of her values, standards, and character traits were rejected by him as undesirable or repugnant. They were no longer perceived as the mother's arbitrary unwillingness to be whatever would please and comfort her child. A secondary object constancy in relation to the mother of the adolescent period became established. The omnipotent mother of the infantile period was superseded by the son's realization of her fallibilities and virtues. In short, she became humanized. Only through regression was it possible for the boy to re-experience the maternal image and institute those corrections and differentiations that effected a neutralization of preoedipal, ambivalent object relations. The psychic reorganization, as described in his case, was subjectively experienced by the boy as a sharp realization of a sense of self, of that awareness, and conviction, best summarized in the phrase of "this is me". The state of consciousness and the subjective feeling, just paraphrased, reflect an emerging differentiation within the ego that is here conceptualized as the second individuation process.

The first exhilaration that comes with the independence from the internalized parent or, more precisely, from the parental object representations is complemented by a depressed affect that accompanies and follows the loss of the internal object. The affect accompanying this object loss has been likened to the state of mourning and to the work of mourning. There remains, normally, a continuity in the relationship to the actual parent after the infantile character of the relationship is given up. The work of the adolescent individuation is related to both these aspects, infantile and contemporary. Both these parental object representations are derived from the same person but at different stages of development. This tends to confuse the relationship of the adolescent to his parent who is experienced partly or wholly as the one of the infantile period. This confusion is worsened whenever the parent participates in the shifting positions of the adolescent and proves unable to maintain his fixed place as an adult vis-à-vis the maturing child. The adolescent disengagement from infantile objects necessitates first their decathexis before libido can again be turned outward in the search of phase-specific object gratifications. We observe in adolescence that object libido—in various degrees, to be sure—is withdrawn from outer and inner objects and is converted into narcissistic libido by being deflected onto the self. This shift from object to self results in the proverbial self-centredness and self-absorption of the adolescent who fancies himself to be independent from the love and hate objects of his childhood. The flooding of the self with narcissistic libido has the effect of self-aggrandizement and an overestimation of the powers of body and mind. This condition affects reality testing adversely. To cite a familiar consequence of this state, I remind you of the frequent automobile accidents of adolescents which occur despite their expert skill and technical knowledge. Should the process of individuation stop at this stage, then we encounter all sorts of narcissistic pathology of which the withdrawal from the object world, the psychotic disorder, represents the gravest impasse.

The internal changes accompanying individuation can be described from the side of the ego as a psychic restructuring during which the decathexis of the parental object representations in the ego brings about a general instability, a sense of insufficiency and of estrangement. In the effort to protect the integrity of the ego organization, a familiar variety of defensive, restitutive, adaptive and maladaptive manoeuvres are set into motion before a new psychic equilibrium is established. We recognize its attainment in a personal and autonomous life style.

At the time when the adolescent process of individuation is in its most vigorous season, deviant, i.e. irrational, erratic, turbulent behaviour is most prominent. Such extreme measures are employed by the adolescent to safeguard psychic structure against regressive dissolution. The adolescent in this state presents the clinician with a most delicate task of discrimination as to the transient or permanent or, simply, as to the pathognomic or normal nature of the respective regressive phenomena. The perplexing ambiguity that clinical assessment has to cope with derives from the fact that a resistance against regression is as much a sign of normal as of abnormal development. It is a sign of abnormal development if resistance against regression precludes a modicum of regression that is essential for the disengagement from early object relations and infantile ego states or, in short, is preconditional for the reorganization of psychic structure. The problem of regression, both ego and drive regression, reverberates through adolescence without let-up. These regressive movements make the attainment of adulthood possible, and they have to be understood in these terms. They also represent the nuclei or the adolescent fixation points around which the failures of the adolescent process become organized. Adolescent disturbances have drawn our attention, almost exclusively, to the regressive symptomatology within the context of drive gratification or to the defensive operations and their sequelae. I submit that resistance against regression is, in equal measure, a cause for concern, when it presents a persistent and unsurmountable roadblock in the course of progressive development.

Resistance against regression can take many forms. One is exemplified in the adolescent's forceful turn towards the outside world, to action and bodily motion. Paradoxically, independence and self-determination in action and in thought tend to become most violent and reckless whenever the regressive pull possesses an inordinate strength. I have observed that children who were extremely clinging and dependent during childhood often resort in adolescence to the reverse attitude, namely, detached distance from the parent at any cost. In doing so they achieve an apparent but illusory victory. In such cases, action and thought are simply determined by the fact that they represent the obverse of expectations, wishes, and opinions of the parent or of their substitutes and representatives in society, such as teacher, policeman, and adults generally or, more abstractly, law, tradition, convention, and order anywhere, in any form, and regardless of their social purpose and meaning. Here again, transient disturbances in the interaction between the adolescent and his environment render them qualitatively different from those that acquire permanency, mould in a definitive fashion the ego's relation to the outside world, and bring the adolescent process to a premature standstill.

Based on our experience with the neurotic child and adult we grew accustomed to concentrate on defences as the major obstacles in the path of normal development. Furthermore, we grew accustomed to think of regression as a psychic process that stands in opposition to progressive development, to drive maturation and to ego differentiation. Adolescence can teach us well that these connotations are limited and limiting. It is true that we are ill prepared to say what, in a regressed state during adolescence, is simply the static resuscitation of the past and what represents the heralding prelude to psychic restructuring. It is reasonable to assume that the adolescent, who surrounds himself with pictures of idolized persons, not only repeats a childhood pattern that once gratified narcissistic needs, but that he simultaneously takes part in a collective experience that makes him an empathic member of his peer group. Sharing the same idols is tantamount to being part of the same family; however, a crucial difference cannot escape us, namely, that the new social matrix at this stage of life promotes the adolescent process through participation in a symbolic, stylized, exclusive, tribal ritual. Regression under these auspices seeks not simply to re-establish the past but to reach the new, the future, via the detour along familiar pathways. A sentence by John Dewey comes to mind here. "The present", he says, "is not just something which comes after the past. . . . It is what life is in leaving the past behind."

The thoughts assembled in this paper have drifted towards a converging goal with the common objective of elucidating the changes in ego organization as they are brought about by drive maturation. It has become convincingly clear from clinical investigations of the adolescent process that both—the task of disengagement from primary objects and the abandonment of infantile ego states—necessitate a return to early phases of development. Only through the re-animation of the infantile emotional involvements and of the concomitant ego positions (fantasies, coping patterns, defensive organization) can the disengagement from internal objects be achieved. This achievement, then, hinges on regression, drive and ego regression, both ushering in, along their course, a multitude of, pragmatically speaking, maladaptive measures. In a paradoxical fashion one might say that progressive development is precluded if regression does not take its proper course at the proper time within the sequential pattern of the adolescent process.

In defining the individuation process as the ego aspect of the regressive task in adolescence, it becomes apparent that the adolescent process constitutes, in essence, a dialectic tension between primitivization and differentiation, between regressive and progressive positions, each drawing its impetus from the other, as well as each rendering the other workable and feasible. The ensuing tension, implicit in this dialectic process, puts an inordinate strain on both ego and drive organization or, rather, on their interaction. This strain is responsible for the many and varied distortions of, as well as failures in, individuation—clinical and subclinical—that we encounter at this age. Much of what appears, at first glance, as defensive in adolescence might, more correctly, be identified as a precondition of progressive development to get under way and to be kept in flux.

It is my hope that the concept of the second individuation will shed light on the structural problems of the adolescent process, because it relates, even synthesizes, such antagonistic trends as regressive primitivization and progressive differentiation, viewing both within their reciprocal influence. In short, what I have endeavoured in this presentation is to make the adolescent paradox explicit and intelligible.

CHAPTER SIX

A note on the crisis of adolescence: from disappointment to conquest

Evelyne Kestemberg

So much has been written and said about adolescence and adolescents[1] in the last decade that I am somewhat afraid of producing a rehash of clichés, however apt some of them may be. Nevertheless, I should like to emphasize here the non-pathological aspect of the adolescent crisis by recalling the truism that adolescence is a time of psychic reorganization induced over a longer or shorter period (of course) by everything that paved the way for it—that is, by every aspect of infantile sexuality and the complex forms of cathexis that have taken place during childhood, as well as by the latency period.

The manner in which the latency period unfolds and its particular colour are in my view vital determinants of the precise form assumed by the onset of adolescence.

Following Freud and many other authors, we have rightly become accustomed to thinking that the prior psychic conflicts—in particular the oedipal ones—are put to sleep during latency, but I

[1]I trust that the authors on whose works I have drawn will forgive me for not quoting them. They themselves, like the reader, will recognize my debt to them; I cannot do justice to each one in a contribution of this length.

am not sure that enough emphasis is being placed on what I see as a very important aspect of the latency period, namely that beneath—or, if you will, concurrently with—that slumber, latency is a time of waiting, and that adolescence must be the crowning glory of the waiting element of the latency period. Hence the puberty that marks the end of and crowns this waiting may, according to whether the expectations are or are not satisfied, be experienced as organizing or disorganizing, or alternatively it may as it were be passed over in silence. There will be no adolescent "crisis" proper, no specific reorganization, experienced as such by the subject at that time. This lack of a critical aspect, if not merely superficial, cannot but bode ill for the subsequent transformation of the psychic apparatus and suggests that the organization that preceded it was deficient.

But if adolescence is openly proclaimed, there are several possibilities, each with different degrees of fertility. Puberty will bring about a sudden or gradual reorganization, accompanied by identity worries and a "jostling" of previous identifications. The awaited adolescence will therefore be experienced by the subject either as profoundly disappointing—that is, the expectations he has nurtured, whether vague or explicit, will have been dashed—or as utterly dazzling, so that he might be tempted to exceed his limitations. In order not to repeat what I and many other authors have already written, let me say that I mean by this that the quintessentially adolescent question "to be or not to be"—that is, the question of *who* to be, which arises with puberty and has latently preceded it—may be experienced as an utter *disappointment*, along the following lines: Well, then, I have reached puberty, I am adolescent, I ought to be different, other social and cultural interests are likely to present themselves, and the world is going to change. But what actually happens? The subject's expectations, more or less conscious plans, and fantasies come face to face with a reality in which the break with the past and the profound changes that had been imagined play no part.

That in itself may give rise to profound disillusionment, putting the subject in conflict not only with his previous identifications—which are in any case highly conflictual at this time—but also with his ideal image of himself. In my view, the immediate fate of the crisis of adolescence will be determined on the level of this idealization, which is always present, although in varying degrees. It seems to me that the adolescent will behave not in accordance with what he was, or with what he is today, or with what his parents are or are not, or with what society does or does not (more often the latter) provide him with, but on the basis of his imaginary and unconscious expectations—of a "new life", as if he had become a new version of himself. Hence the collusion between, on the one hand, the impoverishment of this ideal when confronted with what presents itself to him and, on the other, the persistence of this ideal will allow him either gradually to cut the idealization down to size—a favourable waning of the crisis of adolescence—or conversely to obliterate it, with the result with which we are all familiar—adolescent ennui, which is surely its most worrying aspect. This ennui, gloom, and absence or weakness of cathexes constitute a kind of hyperlatency.

We must in my opinion be very aware of this disappointment, which arouses and carries in its wake the underlying depression that persists in the psychic apparatus throughout life and can only be reinforced by the questioning of identity, including the loss of the dual male and female sexual identity—until, as an extended journey draws to a close, the adolescent, having grown into an adult, reorganizes a psychic bisexuality that has been *reduced* by puberty. I use this word deliberately, for puberty compels the adolescent to have but one sex, to be a man or a woman, and to forfeit the potential to be both—which, as we know, is a very powerful, fertile fantasy that is necessary for mental functioning.

Puberty thus in effect entails the loss of a part of the self, as well as of previous identifications, precisely in proportion as the oedipal conflict can no longer operate at the level of infantile sexuality but is played out with a body capable of fulfilling the oedipal wishes, with the intensely present dangers thereby entailed. It is surely unnecessary to dwell here on the essential and inescapable element of mourning that attaches to this conflict, involving, on the one hand, the murder of the oedipal rival and, on the other, the loss of a certain configuration of the ego ideal and the renunciation of the archaic identifications and primary homosexuality contained therein.

The symptoms accompanying and reflecting this upheaval may be extremely variable and are never in themselves indicative of pathology.

That, to me, is the most difficult thing to understand: the most clamorous manifestations are not the most worrying in terms of the potential psychic organizations of which this crisis is the necessary preliminary.

I should like to illustrate this with a brief clinical vignette. Not long ago I saw, as we all do, an adolescent who, while telling me of a low-level depression that I would rate as trivial, displayed all his conflicts in the way he dressed, which was (if I may put it that way) heterogeneous: some items of his apparel were extraordinarily feminine, while others gave an intensely masculine impression. His behaviour, style, and manner of speaking also betrayed these two modalities, with implicit elements of infantile consonance into the bargain: he was also a lost little boy. That was what struck me most when I saw him. He was gradually led to say that he was not suffering from anything and was suffering from everything; that no one understood him and that he understood everyone; that no one had anything to offer him and yet that it was so simple to hold out a hand to him. His utterances were a constant stream of contradictions, between which he was unable to build bridges and which he could not even perceive as such. All this might appear clamorous, particularly as question marks obviously attached to everything he intended to do. He was in his last year at school; what was he going to do next year? His parents wanted this, he wanted that; no, he did not want anything. Sometimes he would shut himself away in his house, for example in his bedroom, could not bear to be disturbed, and would not speak to anyone, while at the same time complaining that he was being left all by himself and that no one was interested in him; at other times he would effectively yield himself up to a life of roaming. To put the situation in less psychiatric language, he would spend long periods walking or wandering through the streets with a capacity for pleasure, which he did in fact find although he was unable to admit the fact to himself; what he was then really seeking was to rediscover the relative tranquillity of his latency period. These symptoms had greatly troubled his parents, because one day he would go to school and the next day he would not; one day his behaviour would be mocking and demanding, but next day he would be huddled in his bed refusing absolutely everything—yet in spite of his symptoms, he radiated an undiminished living warmth.

I soon realized that a few interviews, in which I would need only to listen to him and show him that he himself was the source of his contradictions—which, as quickly became clear to me, were inherent in his adolescent psychic functioning—would eventually allow him to discover what he wanted to do on the basis of these contradictions themselves; it would then be relatively easy for him to put himself back on track if only he took the time to find himself. And indeed, that is what happened.

The concept of time to which I have just alluded surely merits some brief comments. An extremely archaic stage of psychic organization re-emerges in adolescence, namely the need to have everything, right away, now, as otherwise there is nothing. In other words, the subject is confronted at one and the same time with a momentous project whose fulfilment is greatly idealized and an inability to experience the project as a project and not as immediate fulfilment. Hence the frequent and multiform enactments of adolescents.[2] Perhaps this dimension of time, whereby the project recovers its status both as a project and as a production of the adolescent himself, gives him back his self-esteem and provides him anew with, not an identificatory choice, of which he is incapable at this juncture, but the potential for making an identificatory choice. He will then be able to postpone the immediate satisfaction of wishes that are contradictory and by definition less amenable to fulfilment than ever, and feel that drive impulses may or may not be satisfied on the spot without thereby being extinguished or obliterated. In my view, we have here *the fundamental problem of the period of adolescence, which is that of finding again the time to wait and to fantasize.* It is a matter of reacquiring, in economic terms, a tolerable excitation threshold and, in topographical and dynamic terms,

[2] I am deliberately not dwelling here on delinquency proper or on drug addiction, which are precise aspects of some of these enactments; nor shall I consider in detail the pathological outcomes of the crisis. I do not believe that these aspects call for specific treatment.

a possibility of controlling these excitations without destroying them.

In other words, we have here the *time of conflictuality, a time that is tamed and integrated, allowing the subject to move on from disappointment to conquest*. This conquest may be the clumsy, sensual abandon of Cherubino, in love with every woman, with himself, and even with Figaro, one of whose perspicacious epithets for him is "Narcisetto"; or the bold and passionate hopelessness of Musset's Lorenzaccio; or the blinded, blinding, but nevertheless lucid ardour of the hero of Radiguet's *Le Diable au Corps*; or the cathexis of and impetuous commitment to a political movement or the feverish pursuit of a career, followed later by a return to serenity; or, finally, a temporary vagabond phase, discreetly tinged with romanticism, by which the subject can get the measure of his own strength, the length of his strides, and their good or ill fortune, like the adolescent discussed above, who was composing his "Wanderer" Fantasia in his own way.

As will be seen, the point in all cases is the conquest of self, admittedly through an object, but through one that is in fact barely individualized in its otherness and necessary mainly for its function as a narcissistic "springboard", which, although seemingly remote from the oedipal figures, repeats them unbeknown to the subject, and is also remote from the childhood he seems to thrust away into the distance. The reunion will come later, but the eloquent or torpid prepubertal waiting period will have come to an end, and the former child will have acquired the narcissistic foundations of the adult-to-be. All this, of course, presupposes that the onset and waning of the crisis have taken a favourable course—which, after all, is more often the case than one is inclined to say and write.

Obviously, however, we cannot ignore the opposite situation, in which there has been no conquest and disappointment reigns. I do not wish to describe the pathology of the adolescent and its precursors—nor would this be possible within the bounds of this paper—but shall merely outline some broadly typical cases, which are by no means exhaustive.

For this purpose, let me return to the closing stages of latency and begin by repeating that, expected though it may have been, the acquisition of puberty is *always a surprise*. The child watches out for its signs, observes them, does not believe what he sees, starts to believe and to integrate them, it seems—and suddenly finds himself alien to what he was before (this applies to both sexes). What will he do with this "uncanny" development? I believe that every individual will, if only fleetingly and however repressed it may be, have experienced a moment of glory, followed, in some cases like a billowing wave and in others like an insidious tide, by anxiety. The future will depend on the transformations of this anxiety. There are three possibilities:

1. In some cases the alterations of puberty give rise to almost instantaneous disavowal, obliteration of the change, and immediate or almost immediate filling of the crack—albeit, of course, at the cost of a split in the ego of greater or lesser depth. Everything proceeds as if nothing had happened. The result is a kind of extended hyperlatency, a rejection of the body that is flaunted to a greater or lesser extent or is subtly evident, and, often, a hiatus between the intellect and its source in the drives. The model of anorexia nervosa, which we have described, is an extreme form of this, but there are some that develop more discreetly, although they are substantially similar in their latent content, and still others that are more clamorous, albeit again basically the same in their underlying organization—for example, the delusion-free forms of adult psychosis that we have called "cold psychoses".
2. In another typical case, the alterations of puberty are, by contrast, proclaimed out loud, and an unbridled, promiscuous sexual pragmatism in fact seeks (no less than in the subjects described above, although in a different way) immediately to extinguish novelty and surprise—in other words, to short-circuit conflicts. These are the adolescents I have described elsewhere as presenting a *depression laid bare* and accompanied by inhibition of intellectual or creative activity, who plunge into sexual activism and ultimately find themselves as bare and alone as if they had curled up in bed by themselves. This way of abolishing the unfolding of the crisis, in which the garb of the new person is assumed too quickly (before the new adult person has become established), may itself herald a severe disorder of psychic organization. It eloquently reflects the ego's incapac-

ity to confront anxiety and change, and hence an inability to find a continuity of self within the current discontinuity, as well as a displacement of the erotic cathexis of the body onto the activity of thought.

3. My last typical case is when the breakdown is in effect consummated, the way being paved for adult schizophrenia at the time of adolescence. Here, through the alterations of puberty, the subject discovers his own otherness. He becomes a stranger to himself and to the object, both of which are merged within him. He "gets out of joint", as R. Angelergues aptly puts it, and his thoroughly sexualized thought compels him to reconstruct the world in order to reconstruct himself, without managing to stem the tide of anxiety that constantly disturbs him in his living experience and his body, or, conversely, cruelly immobilizes him in both.

In all these cases, puberty and adolescence will have been *not only critical but also traumatic,* because they will have either devastated the ego or at least disrupted it to such an extent that it is unable to rediscover and use the defence mechanisms that were available to it prior to this new situation, and to resort to, and find a safe haven in, old fantasies. Some will have been able gradually to integrate this trauma—for them, time will have been conquered anew—whereas for others it will prove impossible to overcome and will give rise to severe psychotic reorganizations, whose outcome will remain uncertain for long periods and whose transformation will, as we know, be unpredictable and arduous. Still others will have resorted to suicide as the only possible solution, with its implications of distress coupled with an illusory instant of glory.

Let me conclude with some further brief remarks on latency. I am increasingly discovering a kinship between the latent and hidden sexuality (hidden, that is, from the subject itself) of this period of life, in which the child keeps secret from himself and conceals from others the sexual pleasure he derives from his play—the "obsessional" activities in which we know he indulges being seemingly devoid of all erotism—and the jealous care with which so many adult psychotics hide their delusions or phobias from their own mental functioning.

When all is said and done, while it may be true that everything is prepared in infancy, I believe that it is during the apparent "dissolution" of the Oedipus complex—that is, during latency—that everything is determined, and in adolescence that everything comes together, within the inescapable but in favourable cases temporary discontinuity that puberty and adolescence represent.

This discontinuity is, however, essential. The river must come up against a dam, form whirlpools, and carry its surroundings with it, if it is to get the measure of its own flow, carve out its bed, and proceed on its way to the sea, thereby integrating the new obstacles and oedipal figures that will—perhaps painfully, but always necessarily—enrich it. But if, instead, the dam is bypassed or simply destroyed so that the waters divide, the river will be impoverished, dry up in sterility, or burst its banks as its waters rush away noisily to waste.

CHAPTER SEVEN

The central masturbation fantasy, the final sexual organization, and adolescence

Moses Laufer

For some time now in my analytic work with late adolescents and young adults, I have felt hampered in my ability to understand the meaning of certain clinical material. In a number of instances I found that, although the clinical material of some patients in late adolescence (ages 18 to 21) seemed similar to that of some patients who were young adults (ages 22 to 25 or so), the fact that the patient was either "an adolescent" or a "young adult" seemed fundamentally to affect the meaning of this material. This division between "adolescent" and "young adult" also has determined my diagnostic and prognostic views, as well as my day-to-day technique of work. My first inclination was to explain the difference in meaning by thinking of adolescence as a developmental phase and of young adulthood as a time when structural development is fixed and when the "character" is less amenable to change. As a sweeping definition of the differences between adolescence and young adulthood, this may be correct, but it was not very helpful to me clinically or theoretically. Something much more specific can be added to our understanding of the function of adolescence as part of the developmental process.

Stated in somewhat general terms, my thesis is as follows. Although the resolution of the oedipal conflict means that the main sexual identifications become fixed and that the core of the body image is established at that time, it is only during adolescence that the content of the sexual wishes and the oedipal identifications become integrated into what I believe to be an irreversible sexual identity. During adolescence, oedipal wishes are tested within the context of the person's having physically mature genitals, and a compromise solution (between what is wished for and what can be allowed) is found; it is this compromise solution which, within the variations of normality, defines the person's sexual identity. I therefore see the main developmental function of adolescence in the establishment of the final sexual organization—an organization which, from the point of view of the body representation, must now include the physically mature genitals. The three developmental tasks of adolescence—the change in the relationship to the oedipal objects; the change in the relationship to contemporaries; and the change in the attitude to his own body—can be subsumed under this main developmental function, rather than each being viewed as a separate task in its own right. Once this final sexual organization is established by the end of adolescence, it means that there no longer is a choice for any kind of internal compromise (as may have existed earlier in adolescence). What we then see in young adults, at least in their pathological disorders, is the result of the breakdown in the developmental process that took place in adolescence.

Freud (1905d) begins his essay on "The Transformations of Puberty" as follows: "With the arrival of puberty, changes set in which are destined to give infantile sexual life its final, normal shape" (p. 207). After summarizing his views of infantile sexual life and the pregenital organization of the child, Freud refers to this period as "an important precursor of the subsequent final sexual organization" (p. 234). (See also Chapter 1, this volume.)

In later writings (1923b, 1933a), Freud described the superego as the heir to the Oedipus complex; namely, the resolution of the oedipal conflict results in a new mental structure, the superego, in which the conscience, ideals, and self-criticism become part of a person's internal life and are no longer dependent in the same way on the actual relationship to the parents. In other words, internalization has taken place. We assume that the oedipal identifications play a central role in the person's development through latency and adolescence and actively determine his future relationship both to himself and to other people. I think I summarize Freud's views correctly when I say that he believed that the content of the superego is determined at the time of the resolution of the oedipal conflict, and that any future changes that take place structurally take place within the ego, via post-oedipal identifications or, as in adolescence, via the various transitory identifications that result in the ego's ability to alter its mediating function between the demands of the id and the demands and expectations of the superego (Freud, 1933a; Laufer, 1964). Although the content of the superego may seem to change during adolescence, it is more correct to say that at that time the structures are realigned, and that this realignment takes place via the ego.

When Freud (1905d) describes some of the changes that should take place in puberty—and here he is referring to the subordination of component instincts to the primary of the genitals—he states something that is of special relevance to this paper:

> Just as on any other occasion on which the organism should by rights make new combinations and adjustments leading to complicated mechanisms, here too there are possibilities of pathological disorders if these new arrangements are not carried out. Every pathological disorder of sexual life is rightly to be regarded as an inhibition in development [p. 207]

Later in this paper I shall present clinical material from the analyses of a late adolescent (in treatment from ages 16½ to 21) and a young adult (aged 23) in order to clarify the nature of these new arrangements in adolescence and of the pathological disorders in young adulthood that reflect the breakdown of the developmental process during adolescence. I shall try to show how these new arrangements are tied to the manner in which the content of the central masturbation fantasy is integrated into the person's final sexual organization by the end of adolescence, and how this final sexual organization reflects the way in which the adolescent has been able, by the end of this developmental period, to integrate the physically mature genitals as part of the representation of the body.

The central masturbation fantasy

We assume that, as part of normal development from infancy onward, the person finds means, by using either his own body or an object, of gratifying his instinctual demands. The preoedipal child may have available a whole range of autoerotic activities, games, and fantasies that help to recreate and relive the relationship to the gratifying mother. After the resolution of the Oedipus complex and the internalization of the superego, however, we can no longer refer in the same way to the child's ways of gratifying his instinctual wishes and demands in relation to his first love object, the mother. With the resolution of the Oedipus complex, all regressive satisfactions will be judged by the superego as being either acceptable or not. Moreover, in terms of the future sexual orientation and the "final sexual organization" of the person, the resolution of the Oedipus complex fixes what can best be described as the "central masturbation fantasy"—the fantasy whose content contains the various regressive satisfactions and the main sexual identifications. The fate of the content of this fantasy is of special significance in understanding normal and psychopathological development in adolescence; and the way in which this content forms part of or interferes with development during adolescence can be seen later in the person's adult life.

This central masturbation fantasy is, I believe, a universal phenomenon—its existence or power does not depend on whether or not the child masturbates. During latency the content of this fantasy remains unconscious, but is expressed in a disguised form via daydreams, via the fantasies that accompany masturbation, or via games or make-believe activities and relationships (A. Freud, 1965). Although the latency child's and the preadolescent's reactions to this fantasy and to various forms of autoerotic activity are determined mainly by the reaction of the superego, I believe that only with the physical maturation of the genitals does the content of this fantasy take on a new meaning and make demands on the ego that differ qualitatively from the earlier ones. Although the content of this central masturbation fantasy does not normally alter during adolescence, the fact that it is experienced within the context of physically mature genitals means that the defensive organization is under much greater stress.

The actual ability to impregnate or to become pregnant means normally that the defence against the incestuous wishes (which are contained within the masturbation fantasy) are now tested within a new context; clinically, it is often in this area of functioning that we see the failure of the ego to deal with this new demand. In addition, the oedipal identifications that may have seemed adequate in enabling the latency and preadolescent child to feel secure in his sexual role may prove to be inadequate when tested within the context of genitality. For example, the child's identification with a passive father may seem adequate until adolescence, but then this identification may either hinder the adolescent in his development, or it may be experienced by him as an interference in his efforts to establish his sexual role. It is my impression that much of the acting-out behaviour that we associate with adolescence and often accept as part of normal development can be understood by viewing it as a reflection of the adolescent's efforts to try to find new ways of integrating the central masturbation fantasy. Similarly, some of the breakdowns or temporary psychotic episodes that manifest themselves in adolescence represent the only solution available to the ego (even though it is a pathological solution) in its efforts to find new ways of integrating the content of the central masturbation fantasy within the context of genitality. The clinical material will illustrate some of these points.

"Trial action" in adolescence

In a previous paper (1968) I put forward the view that in adolescence masturbation has the function of helping the ego reorganize itself around the supremacy of genitality. This is normally accomplished by using masturbation and masturbation fantasies as something equivalent to "trial action"—that is, as an autoerotic activity that helps to integrate regressive fantasies as part of the effort to achieve genital dominance. The adolescent's oedipal fantasies are allowed into consciousness, but in a disguised form, and are then normally re-repressed. Some adolescents cannot use masturbation and the accompanying fantasies in this way, but instead experience masturbation or the fantasies as equivalent to failure in repression or as the vehicle for the satisfaction of something perverse or shameful; they cannot use masturbation and the fantasies as a constructive step furthering development to adulthood. I described the internal situation of these adolescents as one of deadlock; they felt that there was no way out of their existing pathology, that nothing was changing, but at the same time they had not yet given in to this internal situation, even though they knew they were stuck in their development.

I now believe that this view of the function of masturbation in adolescence has to be extended. If the thesis that I am putting forward in this paper is correct, it means that the function of masturbation in adolescence is not only that of an action that is experienced within the safety of one's own thoughts, but that it is a way of testing which sexual thoughts, feelings, or gratifications are acceptable to the superego, and which of these are unacceptable and must therefore not be allowed to participate in the establishment of the final sexual organization. However, the problem for the adolescent is not simply which parts of the content of the fantasy, or which regressive wishes in general, are acceptable and which have to be rejected; rather, it is only in adolescence that the person, for the first time in his life, is faced with the adequacy or inadequacy of the defensive organization to help him deal with these problems. He may now feel that he has little ability to defend against certain regressive pulls which, if gratified, would be ego-dystonic, and for which he may be severely punished by the superego. In some adolescents, temporary regression produces acute anxiety because of their fear that they may not be able to re-establish their previous level of functioning; for some adolescents, temporary regression means allowing into consciousness those fantasies and accompanying wishes that represent abnormality but which, at the same time, they may want to gratify (Kramer, 1974; Laufer, 1974).

Late adolescence and young adulthood

As I described earlier, the adolescent will, through trial action, seek ways of finding a compromise answer that will, optimally, enable him to satisfy the wishes contained in the central masturbation fantasy while at the same time obtaining superego approval by satisfying the demands of conscience and the expectations of his ego ideal. This means that, normally, the adolescent must have available some age-appropriate ways of finding gratification and of finding new objects. The reality of having physically mature genitals means that regressive wishes can no longer be allowed the same freedom as previously because now they may threaten the defence organization and bring about superego condemnation.

The problem can be viewed as being a developmental one if genitality remains the main means of gratification. However, as is often the case in pathological development, if the pregenital wishes override genitality, we see severe interference in the adolescent's ability to use masturbation and the accompanying fantasies as trial action. Instead, the sexually mature body is experienced as the source of these regressive wishes, resulting in the need to repudiate it as the means through which gratification can be obtained. The adolescent may, because of the wishes contained in the central masturbation fantasy, feel constantly in danger of giving in to what he both wants and must not allow. In the face of these demands, the adolescent feels passive or, perhaps more correctly, helpless. As a result, he may renounce his ability to control his body or the sensations coming from it.

I believe that the process is different in normal development during this period. However much the adolescent feels in danger of giving in to regressive wishes, he has the unconscious awareness that a choice still exists. If we examine the direction of the libido and the relationships to objects as expressed in the fantasies and especially in the masturbation fantasies, we will find that the libido is object-directed, even though the gratification is of a narcissistic or autoerotic nature; at the same time, the masturbation fantasies of adolescents, especially late adolescents, include the active seeking of a sexual love object. At this point I do not want to examine the nature of the object within the fantasy or the quality of the libidinal gratification; instead, I want to emphasize that part of normal progressive development and part of the trial-action solutions during adolescence have an active quality; that is, the adolescent feels that he is still, at least partially, in charge and in control. This is so whether he imagines himself as the active or the passive one in the fantasy. The important factor from a developmental point of view is that he feels that he (or she) still has the choice to be active or passive within the sexual role. This factor defines the nature of progressive development in adolescence and conveys that the final sexual organization is in the process of being established. It implies that genital as well as pregenital wishes contained in the central masturbation fantasy can still be used actively in the attempt to find an answer. While this may be a compromise answer, it is nevertheless one in which genitality is the final victor.

Something different happens in those adolescents whose defence organization is incapable of warding off the regressive pull of pregenital wishes, and who experience the living out of the central masturbation fantasy mainly as being repetitively overwhelmed. They then experience their sexual body as the source as well as the representative of their abnormality (Laufer, 1968, 1974). These people usually reach a point in their adolescence at which they have a feeling of deadlock (which still contains the fight against giving in); subsequently they have a feeling of giving in, which is then followed by a feeling of surrender. For these adolescents, the predominant wishes remain pregenital, thus precluding the use of masturbation as a trial action; instead, masturbation or sexual gratification from their bodies acts as a constant proof that they have surrendered. In these adolescents, the final sexual organization is established prematurely—prematurely either because the choices are non-existent or because they view choice as an additional threat to an already precarious defence against further regression. What we see, then, especially in young adulthood, is the pathological answer to the conflict that existed during adolescence; it is as if they have accepted that genitality, with regard to both object relationships and gratification, either cannot or must not be attained. They have accepted the fact that there no longer is a choice (Friedman, Glasser, Laufer, Laufer, & Wohl, 1972). I think that such an acceptance signifies the surrender of the body to the mother; it is as if such a young adult has given up genitality in order to avoid the attack from the oedipal parent, while at the same time offering his pregenital body to the mother who first cared for it. The signs pointing to such an outcome exist well before young adulthood, but it is usually only by the end of adolescence that the pathological solution is consolidated into the person's character.

One of the tasks of therapeutic intervention in adolescence is to keep alive this choice; in young adulthood, the task of intervention is to undo the result of the breakdown in the developmental process that took place in adolescence, so that there again exists a choice in the establishment of the final sexual organization (Laufer, 1975a).

Case illustrations

The clinical material is taken from the analyses of two male patients, an adolescent and a young adult, who were both very disturbed people. Although the material I have chosen may represent the extreme of what we meet in analytic work, it highlights the main points I am examining in this paper: the part played by the central masturbation fantasy in the establishment of a final sexual organization by the end of adolescence; and the difference in development and functioning between the adolescent and the young adult. Some of the important differences between these two patients are:

1. The young adult patient feared to recall his adolescence because he could remember it only as a time when he was mad. The adolescent patient also behaved in what may be described as a mad way, but he did not feel that he could not face what had happened.
2. The young adult patient had, during adolescence, experienced a breakdown (Laufer, 1975b)—he had been unable to continue with his studies, had made a number of suicide attempts, and had become seriously dependent on drugs. A similar course was followed by the adolescent—he, too, ended his studies for

a period, became seriously dependent on drugs, and at one point seemed near to death from the drugs, but the masturbation fantasies of this patient showed that his "giving in" differed from that of the young adult.

3. The masturbation fantasies of the young adult patient indicated that he had given up the hope or the expectation of ever finding a sexual love object. The adolescent patient also withdrew from objects, but he had a greater awareness of what was taking place and seemed capable of holding on to the hope that something might still be done to change his life.

THE ADOLESCENT PATIENT

Norman was in analytic treatment (at the Hampstead Child-Therapy Clinic) for a period of 4½ years, from the age of 16½ to 21. Although he first sought help for migraine, depression, and poor attendance at school, it was really his behaviour during masturbation that worried him and which he felt conveyed that he was either mad or a pervert (Laufer, 1968, pp. 131–133). Most often he masturbated in the nude. He liked to have his anus exposed and his buttocks very tensed. Sometimes he hit himself on his back. At other times he crawled about on the floor growling, with the pleasurable idea that somebody might enter his anus; or he masturbated in the living room while his mother was ostensibly asleep in one of the armchairs, placing himself either behind or beside her.

Except for the sudden tragic death of his father when Norman was 12 years old, his history before adolescence sounded uneventful and not unusual. But it soon became obvious that some of his relationships during latency, especially his relationship to the church, foreshadowed the pathological development that became obvious and so worrying during adolescence. When he was alone in the church, he would walk around it with a huge load of books on his back until he was utterly exhausted—a behaviour in which he lived out part of his central masturbation fantasy. The saviour theme and its relation to his masochism and to his need to be humiliated played a very important part in his adolescence.

After Norman had been in treatment for nearly two years, his drug-taking developed into an addiction to methedrine; soon thereafter he stopped coming to treatment. It was during this time that he was near to death. I will not discuss here some of the technical problems encountered, including the technical errors that contributed to the temporary failure in treatment, except to say that it was an error on my part to allow him to give in as he did to the fantasy of being castrated, helpless, a girl. It was obvious throughout his treatment that his castration wish was much greater than his castration fear; the treatment, and later the drug addiction, meant for Norman the giving in to his feminine wish and a perpetuation of the central fantasy of being loved, humiliated, and saved.

I have come across this wish in the treatment of other male adolescents, but the fear of castration and the identification with the oedipal father enabled some of the neurotic adolescents to give up the wish to submit passively to the father and to repress or integrate the derivatives of this passive wish. This process, which can be considered part of normal adolescence, was missing in Norman because his actions, masturbatory as well as others, were always tied to the central masturbation fantasy. None of the regressive behaviour and fantasies ever were separated from this fantasy or subordinated to that of genitality.

He described how, a year or so before he came to treatment, he had dressed up in his mother's slip, pretending that he was a girl. The dressing up was always accompanied by masturbation. His concern about his body, and the need for him or his mother to do things to it, had gone on for a long time. As a child he had worms and his mother would regularly clean his anus. He sometimes thought that the worms had something to do with having been or becoming a girl; the link with a pregnancy fantasy is clear, but it is of interest that when such an interpretation was made, it had no effect whatsoever on him. He recalled that he had been told by his parents that, had he been a girl, he would have been named after his father's favourite sister, and he believed that if he had been a girl he would have been loved more by his father. But to be loved by the father also seemed to contain Norman's wish to be humiliated and punished. Being a girl, having his body cared for, and being humiliated were woven into his masturbation fantasy and were in fact the dominant themes. In the fantasy he was identified with the woman who was being penetrated by the big, powerful man. The feeling of helplessness following masturbation offered him a great deal of satisfaction; he felt cared for, and temporarily he was at one with his mother.

It was during the last year of treatment that I was able to detect a significant change in his masturbation fantasy. Norman began to find it pleasurable to think of having intercourse with one of the girls whom he knew at his college. I had worried that this was, within the transference, another capitulation to me, but gradually he began to test out this fantasy in his real relationships. He started to go out with girls and, after having been with a girl, was able to masturbate with the thought of penetrating her.

To understand what had happened, I need to go back to an earlier period and examine his relationship to his mother at the time he became addicted to methedrine. Just prior to this, his mother was ill with diabetes. Norman began to miss school and spent many hours lying about on the floor. Even though he was temporarily elated when his mother began to get better, his anxiety about her health and his fear that she might die played an important part in his feeling of hopelessness and in his wish to give in and die. He left his school, got a night job, and spent the day high on drugs. He described his feeling after injecting himself with methedrine as "lovely, the penis shrinks, and it's almost impossible to get an erection—but it doesn't matter, because at times like that you don't need a penis." Soon after he left school, he stopped coming to treatment. He stayed away for a month, and returned only after I telephoned and said I wanted him back. Some time later he could tell me how, while he was lying in his room, with syringes by his side, his mother would walk in, talk with him, and behave as if nothing was happening. He would then feel as if nothing mattered, as if nobody cared, so he might as well die. He could also tell me that during the time he was injecting himself, and when he was deciding to leave his school, he had secretly hoped that I would do something to show that I cared for him. When I did not, he felt he might as well give in because nobody was helping him to live. This feeling also contained elements of his relationship to his dead father—it was as if his father, and now I, had withdrawn from him and was forcing him to become a girl.

He was saying that he needed somebody to enable him to respond to the internalized conflict that was there. He could not do it alone partly because the giving in, the dying, and the waiting to be saved were such an integral part of his central masturbation fantasy. He was waiting, I think, either for his mother or myself to take over his body and to help him, but when we behaved as if we did not want his body, he thought that there was no way out of his deadlock.

During the second part of the treatment, various crises arose with which I was able, technically, to deal quite differently than I had in the past. Norman wondered about drugs, and he thought of attacking me in some way by again breaking down. Yet he also began to have different masturbation fantasies, some of which included me. In one version, he would suck my penis and feel loved by me; in another, people were rolled up into small balls—a representation of complete withdrawal, of the wish to suck his own penis, to be totally self-sufficient; in other words, of being both male and female.

It is clear that Norman's breakdown was equivalent to a giving in because of his feeling of hopelessness and his belief that the people who now mattered most, his mother and I, did not care. I think I was finally able to help him because of the fact that the process of treatment enabled him not to give in completely to the pull of the wishes contained in his central masturbation fantasy. My response to him, as well as his mother's great concern for him when she herself improved from the diabetes, helped to create a deadlock—that is, it kept the conflict alive. Treatment did for him what would happen normally during the latter part of adolescence: it aided him in letting the identification with the oedipal father come to the forefront and in utilizing it, both developmentally and defensively, in the establishment of his final sexual organization. Without treatment, the deadlock would have resulted in a giving in; that is, by the end of adolescence or before, his passive wishes to give in, to be a girl, and to have his mother do with his body what she wished would have become integrated into the image of himself. His future is still a precarious one, but without treatment during adolescence—that is, before the establishment of a final sexual organization—the outcome in young adulthood would have been one of perverse sexuality, few if any relationships to people, and possibly a giving in to the point of deciding to die.

THE YOUNG ADULT PATIENT

The second patient, Paul, was in analytic treatment for just over one year, from the age of 23. He did not return to treatment following a summer break, saying that he had now had enough of his mother and myself forcing him to change and that he would organize his life on his own. He was referred to me after he had been asked to leave a psychiatric hospital because he would not accept the hospital rules in general, but mainly because he continued to bring in drugs to the ward.

My knowledge of Paul's history before adolescence is limited. Paul remembered his childhood as a time when everything he did revolved around his mother—playing in the garden, going places with her, and waiting for her to have time for him so that they might go for walks or shopping. At the age of 7 he went to a boarding-school some distance from home. His parents sent him there because his older brother was there and because they wanted him to have a good education. Although he was very unhappy for a time, he "got used to it". He made some friends, but most of the time he spent alone. The picture he had of that period was of being teased and bullied, crying in his room, waiting for his parents to visit, and dreading the time when the visit would end. At the age of 18, still at the boarding-school, he attempted suicide and was admitted to the local mental hospital, where he stayed for some months. During this time he wrote his exams for university entrance and passed them well. The suicide attempt was not taken seriously either by his family or by himself. He went to the university, where after a few weeks he made another suicide attempt, and then left the university. He did nothing for some months, but during this time he began to smoke a great deal of marijuana, which he has continued to do up to the present.

At the boarding-school he had begun to feel that something was wrong with his thoughts. The only thing that could comfort him during his periods of despair and emptiness was his teddy, which he had had since early childhood. He still had it, and it remained important to him. At the school as well as now he would hug it close to him, and this would help to remove the empty hole which he felt existed inside his chest. At school he had begun to feel that anything was better than having nobody to love him, and he still believed that it was this that made him think that a homosexual relationship was at least a way of being held and cared for. At school he had a close relationship with one boy of his own age; they masturbated each other, and Paul let his anus be investigated, "but that was all". He recalled it as something that he did not like much, "but it was better than crying". Following the suicide attempt at university (and leaving the university), he met a man a few years older than himself, with whom he had a homosexual relationship. This included fellatio, anal intercourse, and Paul being tied to a bed after which the man masturbated him. Paul said that he did not mind this because it was at least somebody being interested in him.

During the period of the treatment, and for some time prior to it, he had almost no contact with his parents. He believed that all they wanted was to get him to conform and to be a good son. He repeatedly stated that he did not care what happened to either parent, but at the same time he waited anxiously for a weekly letter from his mother; if it came a day late, he would be furious, saying that this was a confirmation that she did not care. For much of the year in treatment, he was unable to keep a job because of his difficulty in getting up in the morning. He used to go to sleep between 3 and 7 in the morning, having spent most of the night either drinking or smoking hash. He told me that as a child he was terrified of the dark and needed his mother to be with him when he went to bed. When she left the room, he would have to hug his teddy, otherwise he was frightened that something might happen to him. At boarding-school this was easier to cope with because there were other boys in the room and he could feel safe with them; but he still needed his teddy in bed. Now, he had to drink each night or smoke hash until he was unaware of where or who he was. This was the only activity that enabled him to put out of action that part of his mind which said that he was bad or dirty. If he lay in bed at night and was not drunk or high on drugs, part of his mind would attack him and say he was useless and bad. But during the day he was not aware of this part of his mind, so long as he could feel that his mind and his body were under control—that is, so long as he felt nearly dead most of the day. He spent much of his day looking for places to buy marijuana, wandering the streets, or visiting people whom he had met at the hospital and who would then feed him and care for him.

His masturbation activity and fantasy had continued without much change from his early adolescence onward. He would first drink or smoke hash; then he would lie on the floor in the dark, imagining somebody doing something to him (he could not be sure what). He would then switch on the light and put on his mother's, and more recently his aunt's, dress. He would then undress, hit his back or buttocks, and masturbate. He could not be sure who was hitting him. This made him feel good because the alcohol, the masturbation, and the hitting deadened him for the rest of the day. The nearest he got to describing what fantasy was active during the time he was hitting himself was to say that he felt somebody was caring for him. His aunt appeared in the fantasy a few times, but he had no idea what she was doing.

During the period of treatment it was extremely difficult to reconstruct the time in adolescence when he felt that his world had collapsed and when he began to believe that nothing could be changed. It was as if the experience of the breakdown—exemplified by his suicide attempt and his admission to the mental hospital—was traumatic inasmuch as he felt completely overwhelmed by internal forces without having any ability at that time to cope with them (Laufer, 1974, 1975a). Nor did he feel that he could turn to the outside world for help in dealing with these forces. All he could say about this time was that it was lonely and that he did not care whether he lived or not. He wanted to die, he said, when he felt sure that his mad thoughts and his activity during masturbation would never change. Internally, both during the time of his breakdown in adolescence as well as now, he felt that nothing mattered, that there was nothing he could do about his sexual life and about his relationships to other people, and that if he died it simply was "too bad".

Part of my initial task in treatment was to try to reawaken a feeling of wanting or needing people. For a while he felt that I was the only person he could trust, and that it was only in treatment that he could risk showing the extent of his despair. He could, for the first time in years, talk about and begin to feel the severe depression and the feeling of emptiness underlying his present behaviour. But this was something much too painful to experience—he said that he had begun to dread coming to see me, even though he liked me, because I talked to him about the things that he had wanted to forget and which he had begun to believe did not matter any longer. He now thought of me as the person who might make him remember the most terrible time in his life (referring both to the time he went to boarding-school and the time in his adolescence when he felt he was becoming a pervert; worst of all was the feeling that nobody cared what happened to him at either time).

When he felt that I cared for him, he was able to find work for a while, and he could begin to express some annoyance both with himself for being so dependent on drugs and with the drug-pushers who he felt were living off his weakness. He could even begin to feel that he missed me during the holiday breaks. But at the same time he was convinced that the treatment was not really doing anything to help him change his attitude to his body and to his penis. It was as if the beginning longing for people emphasized for him the extent to which he had, from the time of his breakdown in adolescence, tried to find ways of excluding any objects from his sexual life. His present sexual life, which consisted mainly of masturbation, lying in bed with his teddy, or caressing his body, contained the repetitive living out of his central masturbation fantasy and the defence against the anxiety aroused if he felt dependent on anybody. Via the drugs, his teddy, the benefits from the social security office, and his aunt, he could feel that the image of himself as somebody with a non-functioning penis did not matter; instead, to be cared for as he now was perpetuated the idea that he had successfully disowned his sexual body and that he had now given in completely. (His beating fantasy represented his relationship to the oedipal father; the further regression which was precipitated by the living out of this fantasy represented the surrender of his body to the preoedipal mother.)

From Paul's description of his actions and thoughts during masturbation, it seemed that his final sexual organization became established at the time of the breakdown in adolescence; very little had changed in his life since that time. There was no change at all in his masturbation fantasies; unaltered, they had become integrated into his character. It was as if his whole life now was a repetitive living out of his masturbation fantasy. Moreover, he seemed to feel compelled to live his life in a very specific way. The developmental possibilities that may have existed during adolescence were destroyed, I believe, at the time of the breakdown.

Some implications for diagnosis, prognosis, and treatment

If it is a psychological fact that a person's final sexual organization is established by the end of adolescence, a correct diagnosis and treatment in adolescence can be important for the whole future life of that person. There are people who put forward the view that the period of adolescence itself is a time when treatment, especially intensive treatment, is contraindicated. The views I have put forward in this paper have contained in them the reasons why I think that such a belief is incorrect. I would say that if the developmental process in adolescence either is seriously interfered with by internalized conflict or has stopped as the result of a breakdown in functioning, then treatment is not only indicated but urgent (Laufer, 1975b). It is urgent because we may still be able to aid progressive development and help the adolescent in his effort to integrate genital functioning into his final sexual organization. There are some adolescents who are prone to severe and quick regression, and who are in danger of organizing their lives, as did Paul, almost totally around the living out of their central masturbation fantasy. As I have tried to show in the clinical material of Norman and Paul, prognostically the signs for future pathology are serious when a breakdown occurs which halts the developmental process or, more seriously, which is experienced as a traumatic episode.

On the basis of these considerations, some specific diagnostic criteria for late adolescence and young adulthood can be defined. We should be especially concerned with (1) whether the libido is still object-directed, or whether there are signs of withdrawal from objects; (2) whether the adolescent's relationship to his body shows an active ability to integrate the physically mature genitals, or whether there are signs of his giving in and disowning his sexual body; (3) whether the thoughts and behaviour show some detachment from the central masturbation fantasy, or whether this fantasy is constantly being repeated in thought and behaviour. One of the diagnostic problems, however, is that these factors frequently become clear only in treatment. The criteria can nevertheless help us be more specific in our judgement.

With young adults there are additional important items, both diagnostically and therapeutically, which need to be taken into account. Care needs to be taken, in work with young adults, not to consider behaviour or thought that is characteristic of adolescence as a sign either of some transitory interference in development or of "prolonged adolescence" (Bernfeld, 1923; Blos, 1954)—a description with which I take issue both clinically and theoretically. Instead, such behaviour indicates that the person was stuck in his development in adolescence, and that what we now see is the pathological solution of the earlier conflict. I would say, from my experience in treatment, that the move from adolescence into young adulthood occurs at about the age of 21. Around that time a person's way of dealing with anxiety becomes much more predictable, the quality of his object relationships is set, and the channels for libidinal gratification have become much more specific.

A breakdown in adolescence leaves some young adults with a feeling of having been mad, and their reality testing having been damaged; this was so with my patient Paul. Treatment has to enable these young adults to understand and work through what they experienced as a trauma in their adolescence. This involves working through what led to the breakdown and the accompanying feeling of having been mad in some way. Even with less disturbed adult patients than Paul, the reconstruction and the working through of their adolescence are important because this was the time in their lives when the internalized conflicts and the interferences that existed in the establishment of their final sexual organization resulted in a great deal of mental pain. Some of my young adult and adult patients have much difficulty in recalling their adolescence; it is for them mainly a time that frightened them, and a time they do not want to remember. Yet when patients are able to understand what happened during that period, it also enables them to make more affective sense of their earlier lives.

CHAPTER EIGHT

The pubertal, its sources and fate

Philippe Gutton

The processes of adolescence are expressed through normal and/or pathological phenomena and may be classified as falling into the following three groups: (1) psychic transformations associated with puberty; (2) genital object choice and identity; and (3) the referential or subject-related system whereby these choices are elaborated (references and the referent).

Psychic transformations associated with puberty: the pubertal

Puberty is to the body what the pubertal is to the psyche. Human sexuality develops in two phases, separated by the latency period (Freud, 1905d), but there is also an "approximation of the child's sexual life to that of the adult" (Freud, 1923e, p. 142). All our studies focus on that approximation. Puberty necessarily entails a discontinuity that cannot be bypassed or postponed. To disregard it would be a self-mutilation. The emergence of the second, genital, sexual differentiation comes as a surprise to the child, who cannot possibly have anticipated it and can have only "a premonition of what are later to be the final and normal sexual aims" (Freud, 1919e, p. 187). "It is not until development has reached its completion at puberty that the sexual polarity coincides with *male* and *female*" (Freud, 1923e, p. 145).

The gradual process of genital differentiation results from the complementarity of the sexes that characterizes libidinal functioning at puberty. It is worth defining the concept of complementarity, which does not appear in *The Language of Psychoanalysis* (Laplanche & Pontalis, 1967), is not used by Freud, and is understood on the basis of amphimixis (Ferenczi, 1924). It reflects a matching of organs along the same lines as the pair "erotogenic zone/part-object" (which psychoanalysis sees in terms of the interactive functioning of the breast and the baby's mouth). When the libido comes to centre qualitatively and quantitatively on the genital zone, infantile autoerotism is at an end, and the commitment to heterosexuality has been made: the male organ is "experienced" in the presence of the female organ, whether present or hallucinated, and vice versa. This intimate interaction is expressed in an initially undifferentiated primary affect or experience in which the representations will allow the two organs to be differentiated. Otherness is obviously not acknowledged in this type of functioning. At this regressive relational level, the partners' interaction may be said to be guided by what the nineteenth-century biologists called the "intuition of instinct". This trust in action may be regarded as the source of the enactment that is characteristic of adolescent pathology. "Now, however, a new sexual aim appears" (Freud, 1905d, p. 207). The sexual drive draws closer to its biological sources, and its transformation is manifested in the capacity for fecundation and the model of the pleasure principle (orgasm). This return of the drive to the somatic level takes the genital to its archaic pubertal source. The complementarity of the sexes must be distinguished from the characteristic pairs of opposites of infantile psychic bisexuality—in particular, passive/active and seduced/seducer. Infantile sexual theories (Freud, 1923e) are of course at variance with genital sexuality, which is symbolized by the complementarity of the sexes. In these theories, the infantile genital organization "consists in the fact that, for both sexes, only one genital, namely the male one, comes into account. What is present, therefore, is not a primacy of the genitals, but a primacy of the *phallus*" (p. 142). The phallus—the signifier of the paternal function—is the "token of the right sex"[1]: infantile sexuality is male. The difference between the sexes is governed by the degree to which the phallic signifier is present, on a scale extending from "phallic" at one end to "castrated" at the other. Pubertal pressure has the aim of separating phallus and penis. Once the penis has been liberated from its phallic significance, the female sex[2] is revealed in the place where phallic castration had been expected.

The "new sexual aim" (Freud, 1905d, p. 207) has to be experienced through a part-object. To find the aim of the drive means being induced to represent the object of the drive. The part-object of the complementarity of the sexes, in close proximity to its biological origins, is an incentive to representation. What transforms this interaction between experienced part-objects into intersubjectivity? What allows the child to interpret what he feels in a new and unexpected way? This psychic work, which takes the experiences of puberty as its starting point, may be likened to the dream work operating on latent thoughts (day's residues or internal and external somatic stimuli). The past offers itself to provide meanings, and to transform what is as yet a jumble of experience into words and behaviour. The sensual current "never fails, apparently, to follow the earlier paths and to cathect the objects of the primary infantile choice with quotas of libido that are now far stronger" (Freud, 1912d, p. 181). These objects are the oedipal figures that stimulate the subject to revive and revisit the infantile Oedipus complex. The hallucinated other sex (as the baby hallucinates the nipple) looks for its place in the person of the incestuous parent. The violence of the pubertal drives is connected less with the increase in somatic energy levels than with this translation into incestuous and parricidal representations. The pubertal capacity for representation may even be regarded as functioning as a pro-

[1][*Translator's note*: This term (*indice du bon sexe* in French) is due to J. Laplanche. Sex here refers to both anatomy and function (i.e. perception and representation).]

[2][*Translator's note*: In the sense of the previous note.]

tective shield against stimuli where genital experiences are concerned. Puberty makes heavy demands on the capacity to fantasize. As we know (Mâle, 1982), the failure of this capacity gives rise to ennui, which is deemed to be a defence and an indication of potential psychosis. Owing to his history, the child at puberty finds himself strangely subjected to the desire of the parental object. The pubertal is quite the antithesis of a movement of separation. A force directed against separation fuels the child's frenzy towards his parents. It is important to realize that the pubertal primal discovery of the new "sexual aim" is "diverted" by its very mental image: sexuality may have found its aim, but it has not found an appropriate object.

The concept of the *pubertal scene* is used in our research as a metaphor to exemplify these internal and external processes. On the basis of what may be called the new pubertal archaic, it contains and elaborates past infantile scenes, which can now undergo metonymic transformation. "The child at puberty suffers from pubertal scenes", as I once put it (Gutton, 1991). These scenes feature the leading man or lady, namely the child, whose erotogenic body is centred on the aroused genital organs, as well as the parental figures of incest and its prohibition. Here the infantile is neither forgotten nor remembered, but repeated. Representations of actions are dispensed with, as in primary functioning. In this sense, the pubertal scene is implicitly enacted. The issue of the body in fact arises on two levels: that discussed above, and that of its incestuous meaning. Moses and Eglé Laufer (1984) have clearly demonstrated the adolescent's dialectically opposed efforts to externalize the body, which is experienced as seducing or persecuting, and to internalize it in the constitution of his genital identity. The interactive conceptualization of the pubertal scene is in our view important; it has elements both of the child's psychic transformations and of what I have called *the pubertal of the parents*—that is to say, the profound changes undergone by the parents at the time of their child's puberty, involving not so much a resurgence of their memories as processes from their own adolescence. As in the Oedipus story, which generation is seducing which, and which generation is attacking which? The pubertal scene is not a fantasy but is already an implicit or explicit behaviour in which the adolescent secretly knows that his oedipal representations have their counterparts in his parents. This knowledge becomes absolute conviction only in psychosis. The pubertal is traumatic if the adolescent's unconscious desire encounters a complementary desire in one of his parents, as for example in consummated incest.

The pubertal differs from the infantile in two respects. First, the asymmetry of the Oedipus complex at puberty decisively favours heterosexuality. Infantile homosexuality is normally decathected, sublimated, and repressed, but it may sometimes be desired and projected. If it exerts excessive pressure, this will impede pubertal development and contribute to pathology. Second, incest falls within the category of the possible but is blocked by prohibition (this is the paradox arising at the end of the infantile state of incomplete development). The choice of object is made between possibility and incestuous prohibition, between action and dream (Ladame, 1991).

The linchpin of the change represented by adolescence is the pubertal scene—or, more precisely, the latter's fundamental mismatch between internal and external reality. This scene demands an elaboration based on the use of cathected objects.

The pubertal scene plunges the infantile oedipal organizations—the agencies of Freud's second topography—into crisis. The superego, as both censorship and ego ideal, proves substantially incapable of repressing the incestuous and parricidal representations and of offering an identificatory model, confronted as it is with not only a quantitative and qualitative modification (the end of the stage of incomplete development) but also a considerable external parental contribution (seduction and aggression). Reality testing, established by the processes of latency, finds itself in difficulties. The ego, as the locus of the reality principle, now lacks the buttressing of infantile biological immaturity. We have emphasized the anti-narcissism of the pubertal scene. The childhood alliance between ego and superego forged during latency cannot continue. Whereas during childhood prohibition and impossibility were linked—that is, negotiated—puberty separates them, so that any prohibition potentially gives rise to frustration or paranoid projection. The alliance is likely to be broken asunder, so that adaptations are necessary in order to shore up the agencies on which the subject's referential system is based.

The adolescent crisis, whether normal or pathological, is a quest for solutions to the problem of guaranteeing a continuous sense of existence while at the same time integrating the novelty of puberty. This integration presupposes the adaptation and consolidation of the agencies of the second topography. A failure here takes the form of a breakdown in the subject's history along the lines described by Moses and Eglé Laufer. The ego's response to the pubertal attack is a pathological split.

Frightened by the pleasure-mediated convergence between his now pubertal body and the pubertal positions of the parents, the adolescent may find himself at the mercy of an unsuspected representation of violence that the prohibition of incest may prove unable to control. At this point, on

> the one hand, with the help of certain mechanisms he rejects reality and refuses to accept any prohibition; on the other hand, in the same breath he recognizes the danger of reality, takes over the fear of that danger as a pathological symptom and tries subsequently to divest himself of the fear. [Freud, 1940e (1938), p. 275]

That is the principle of pubertal psychosis, a term I have previously used to reflect the historico-dynamic point of view. What is specific to such a state in puberty is the role of the genital body, the symbol of the "danger of reality", as seducer and persecutor, coddled (hypochondria) and hated (attempted suicide), stimulated and accused. The correct clinical approach is, as for borderlines in particular, addiction in the broad sense (which may or may not involve drugs), and fetishistic and perverse organizations, whether temporary or permanent. In more severe cases, the collapse of the ego corresponds to outright psychosis.

The elaboration I have termed *"adolescens"* (Gutton, 1996) is called for as the transformations of puberty progressively take place. The *"adolescens"* deals with these transformations in accordance with their demands. It is a transference that results from the need for, or necessity of, transferring the pubertal, with whose transmissive force the child is imbued. This transference arises out of the pubertal deadlock and the need to become a subject. It is made up (Freud, 1900a) of two components that are examined below: the content of the displacement, and the addressee of this content.

The pubertal is not merely a repetition of the infantile, because it introduces a fundamental change. The theory of *Nachträglichkeit*[3]—remembering—constructs the choices of identity and of genital objects in accordance with such a model. In the analytic session, the result is a transference onto words. The addressee of this transaction receives its message. That third party, or Other—the "parental transference object" (Gutton, 1996)—is at once the locus of resistance and the engine of the transference processes. It lies at the heart of the referential system of the adolescent process of becoming-a-subject.[4]

Genital object choice

Even if a new sexual aim has appeared in the pubertal, the drive has not yet found potentially appropriate objects. The sensual current

> runs up against the obstacles that have been erected in the meantime by the barrier against incest; consequently it will make efforts to pass on from these objects which are unsuitable in reality, and find a way as soon as possible to other, extraneous objects with which a real sexual life may be carried on. [Freud, 1912d, p. 181]

The orientation towards these new "*extraneous objects* with which a real sexual life may be carried on", and in respect of which the adolescent may hope to achieve equilibrium between narcissism and the drives, calls for an unconscious transference of the puber-

---

[3][*Translator's note*: This is the word originally used by Freud and translated by Strachey as "deferred action", a rendering that is now considered controversial because, unlike the French equivalent *après-coup*, it does not give sufficient weight to the idea of retroactive revision.]

[4][*Translator's note*: See note regarding "becoming-a-subject", Chapter 9.]

tal representations. These objects will not be created (as in the classical view) "in accordance with the prototype (image) of the infantile object", but will be modelled on and have the characteristics of the pubertal objects. The process is that of associative thought: the tactic I have called *"adolescens"* is deployed as it were aimlessly. This formulation is intended to stress the idea that the prior psychic work on the pubertal material combines sublimation and idealization. Against this necessary background (its absence carries a risk of pathology), such "aimless" construction presupposes that the pubertal scenes are first erased and that their traits and affinities are then re-found in new objects. Love experiences, in particular when shared, as well as their break-up, are prime examples of the confrontation between, on the one hand, objects and parental images and, on the other, objects and new images. Through his capacity to stage love scenarios, the adolescent informs us that he is burying the pubertal scene while at the same time organizing it. A void is required between the burial and the resurgence, otherwise the new love cathexes will be experienced as dangerous. But if the void is excessive, we have the characteristic ennui of adolescent psychopathology. Resistance within the processes of adolescence is signalled by difficulties in these normal and abnormal carry-overs from the pubertal. As a secret source-object, the pubertal scene is metamorphosed into an adolescent scene following the subterranean transference in which the parental representations undergo repression and the parental objects a disengagement.

What is repressed are the figures of the pubertal scene. More precisely, whereas the superego admittedly represses the representations, the pubertal scene also includes perceptions, or even perceptual illusions bordering on hallucination, which call for a process of negative hallucination (Green, 1993). The representations of the new love objects benefit from a return of this repressed. The state of being in love, which is comparable in this respect to the sense of the uncanny, could thus be interpreted as a "parapraxis". Inherent in it is the paradox that the components of the pubertal scene must remain sufficiently unrecognized, whereas the cathexis of the wish depends on the very characteristics of their representations (which are displaced and condensed). Object choice and genital differentiation result from the resolution of the contradiction. I have previously called this process of deconstruction–reconstruction the *adolescent neurosis of development*. Its oedipal structure reflects a psychic process that links two sets of components: first the infantile neurosis, which is recognized within it retrospectively (Lebovici, 1980) by its structural carry-overs and its material, and, second, the transformations of puberty. Three levels are distinguishable between the adolescent neurosis and the infantile neurosis:

1. a simple repetition modelled on the infantile neurosis, with quantitative drive reinforcement
2. a "complicated transformation" or "elaborative repetition", which is a memory effect akin to *Nachträglichkeit:*

   > people's "childhood memories" are only consolidated at a later period, usually at the age of puberty; and . . . this involves a complicated process of remodelling, analogous in every way to the process by which a nation constructs legends about its early history. [Freud, 1909d, p. 206 n.1]

3. a "reshuffling" of objects—the Oedipus complex is uncompleted because the oedipal structure is not synchronized with biological maturation; as a result the

   > infantile object-choice was only a feeble one, but it was a prelude, pointing the direction for the object-choice at puberty. . . . From this time onwards, the human individual has to devote himself to the great task of detaching himself from his parents. . . . For the son this task consists in detaching his libidinal wishes from his mother and employing them for the choice of a real outside love-object. [Freud, 1916–1917, Lecture 21, p. 336f]

   The idea is pursued in this interpretation of the Wolf Man's development (Freud, 1918b):

   > This [sensual, masculine] current had to struggle against the inhibitions that were derived from its infantile neurosis. There had been a violent revulsion in the direction of women, and he had thus won his way to complete masculinity. From that time forward he retained women as his sexual object; but he did not enjoy this possession, for a

> powerful, and now entirely unconscious, inclination towards men . . . was constantly drawing him away from his female objects. . . . [Freud, 1918b, p.117f]

So the pubertal is an organizing factor whose aim is the construction of the adolescent neurosis, which translates the conflicts into representations in the form of *adolescent fantasy scenes*. Here is the origin of the resistances of adolescence and the concomitant pathological neurotic models of anxiety, conversion, and phobia. The representations of potentially appropriate objects in sexual and emotional life are differentiated here. These scenarios are like photographic negatives of what is and will be revealed in love experiences and in both adolescent and adult psychoanalytic transferences.

Disengagement mechanisms (Lagache, 1958) are applied to the pubertal parental objects. They reconstruct the (family) setting within which the adolescent neurosis of development is organized. Two such mechanisms may be distinguished:

1. *Processes of obsolescence.* These signal parental disincarnation or disembodiedness in the pubertal scenes, amounting to a release from parental mastery. The adolescent thereby relinquishes the incestuous link (whether at imago or reality level) between his body and the parental body (each as represented in the pubertal scene). The important point is idealization of the parental object. This idealization is hardly conceivable without interactivity—that is, obsolescence of the parents' pubertal.
2. *Mourning work.* Failing obsolescence of the pubertal object, that object must be lost. This mourning work re-creates substitutive representations that retain the traces of the parental objects. However, the infantile parental object has already been lost many times over: at the time of the pubertal archaic violence that swept away the post-oedipal tenderness of latency; at the time of transition from the genital experience and part-objects to the incestuous whole object; and at the time of the pubertal failure due to the prohibition of incest. The mourning state is reflected in the attempt to preserve the physical presence of the parents and in the impression of being physically separate from them even when they are present. The term

"anticipated mourning work" is preferable where this process takes place in the presence of the real parents.

The disengagement mechanism that demands object loss is much more drastic and less silent than obsolescence. While some adolescents separate easily, most carry with them a sense of loss, a lack commensurate with their adolescent acquisitions and love life. "If the child is to become adult, then this move is achieved over the dead body of an adult" (Winnicott, 1971). The capacity to transfer love from the parental objects to new objects compensates for the loss of the former entailed by the cathecting of the latter. Such a fate indicates that obsolescence has failed and impedes the organization of the adolescent neurosis of development. Adolescent development comes virtually to a halt; puberty seems to give rise to a depressive mood, a sense of impotence and non-adaptation to the world, a void in thought: where has the object gone? This depressive mood must be clearly distinguishable from a breakdown in the subject's history if the two phenomena are to be identifiable when present in combination in one and the same adolescent. The depressive believes that he can heal his suffering by working through it internally. He is not driven to enact. The depressive's terror is of no longer being able to represent. In breakdown, however, the only stage upon which the representations can organize themselves while at the same time disappearing is that of the body in action: the adolescent is alone with his body (Laufer & Laufer, 1984).

References and the referent

The transference of the representations of the parental objects onto "extraneous" love objects is directed towards a transference object, an Other, or referent, whose status is in every respect comparable to the psychoanalyst in analytic therapy—that is, as the organizing point of life. This follows if the "*Adolescent* Processes" (Gutton, 1996) are seen as analogous to those of analysis ("what analysis achieves for neurotics is nothing other than what normal people bring about for themselves without its help" [Freud, 1937c, p. 225]). The addressee has the dual status of an internal interlocutor and a third party. This mixed conceptualization of the transference object is, in my view, important, because that object not only takes part in the subject's intimate, secret dialogue and is included in his daytime and nocturnal fantasy life, but it also has external, incarnate characteristics. The relationship is therefore characterized by intersubjectivity, by a genuine interdependence between the subject engaged in his adolescence and his Other. Adolescence must be a shareable and shared experience if it is to be a familiar construction. The transference object is an object that is already there (in Winnicott's sense), in the process of construction and reconstruction, present in the environment, yet elected by the adolescent himself. It is permanent and continuous in its historicity, while at the same time modifiable as development proceeds, so that the subject can look at his own evolution and on the past, present, and future.

I call this referent the *parental transference object*. It is the parental Other, both internal and external, not an object of (pubertal) desire, not a symmetrical double (adolescent narcissism), and not a mere projection of the ego and superego agencies or of the infantile parental imagos, but instead a psychic construction, both mutable and immutable, made up of these ingredients and having a substrate of flesh. While able to observe the ego as an object, it is also a witness to the process of becoming-a-subject. It buttresses the subject's narcissism at all times as well as being his conscience, the measure of the discrepancy between the actual and the ideal ego. This parental transference object serves as a "committed interpreter" (Aulagnier), who interprets not the adolescent and his actions, acts, and words, but his very transferences. This intersubjectivity is the space-time in which the adolescent's transference and the parental object's countertransference are organized, the fruit of a two-fold tendency both towards and against the other. It is in effect a process of mutual translation or construction, of elaborative mutual activity: parents and adolescents "speak the language of the pubertal", or more precisely that of the potential blockages to its working through, and they comment on and moderate this language.

The parental transference object is constructed from the pubertal objects by an unconscious psychic process combining sublimation and obsolescence. Stemming as it does from the real and imaginary parents, it gives rise to the errors about the person stated by Freud to occur in analysis. It is seen as an object of desire, and the adolescent believes himself to be sexually enslaved to it or neglected, humiliated, or offended by it. It may be granted power (parental grandiosity)—the power to seduce, frustrate, or persecute. A dialectical opposition arises between the third party and the charms of its image or its reality. A good example of this situation is to be found in Blos (1984), who contrasts the homoerotic attachment to the father with the capacity for identification and superego construction during adolescence.

Which aspects of the parental transference construction may be—somewhat reductively—attributed more to the maternal and which more to the paternal functions (both resulting from the transformations of puberty)? The interactive basis of the pubertal scene is in effect a primal narcissistic unity (akin to the mother–baby dyad), which rediscovers, re-actualizes, and reuses the link with the primordial maternal position, the "good-enough mother", as it were the official container of the alpha function (Bion, 1962). The reconstruction of narcissism after its injury by the pubertal is a job for two parties. The antithesis between narcissism and pubertal scenes is thus dialectical, involving both attack and support.

I have called the object assigned the function of compromise under the aegis of the ego the *pubertal narcissistic* object. This approach follows from the work of Kestemberg and takes account of the narcissistic negotiations demanded by the violence of the object. It is also inherent in the concept of the "widened psychic space" (Jeammet, 1980). The pubertal narcissistic object corresponds to a complex experience. Its functioning by projective and introjective identification does not exceed the bounds of representation of the physical presence of the (maternal) object. It is itself the creator of adolescent identifications and fantasy activity.

Let us now return to the referent. Without here discussing the theory of the role of the third party in psychic processes, we may distinguish three modes of functioning that may be present in the development of each adolescent:

1. The certainty of genital identity presupposes an internalization of the third-party function. This function has been acknowledged and replaces the parental transference object. The adolescent operates in accordance with an identificatory project. Following the pubertal attack on the superego, the latter is reconstructed after a certain transaction time as both censorship and ego ideal. It is adapted to the new situation. This functioning substantially corresponds to the end of adolescence or, if you will, the end of an analysis.
2. Where the identificatory conviction is inadequate, it needs the support of a good-enough paternal image. This is the mask then donned by the parental transference object. The now fragile superego needs to be buttressed by the Other in order to negotiate adolescence and to acquire the means to resume its functions. In this process, it is important to distinguish the role of internal representation from that of the physical presence, or incarnation, of the paternal function (the imaginary and the real father). In order to be idealized, this third object may generate an erotico-aggressive fascination. In the adolescent transaction, it buttresses the inadequate functioning of the superego, like St Christopher carrying the Infant Jesus, and, in particular, it moulds that agency in a form ensuring that it can operate effectively in the future. By its originality it enables and implements change, as well as preventing a breakdown in the subject's history. In its absence, the novelty of puberty would fade away. In most societies the reference object is situated exogamously in a group outside family control. Because it is therefore not the paternal third object, it can be embodied in the external person of a leader, teacher, or friend. In this commonplace situation, a conflict may arise between the parental object and a given reference object, when the cathexis of one as referent entails the de-idealization of the other (and vice versa). The state of being in love is an interesting example. In this state the partners share the attraction stemming from the drive as well as a common referential basis, so that one partner's ego ideal has the same aspirations as the other's. Love performs a mutative function in adolescent development owing to this referential commonality. In analysis, the adolescent transference is to be

understood in terms of the parental transference object and of negotiation between substitution and rivalry. Its two extremes are excess (massive transference), where the transference object becomes utterly grandiose, and deficiency, where the hyper-cathected parents take centre stage and prevent any exogamous third-party intervention.

3. The adolescent's reference in the third mode of functioning is ideology (religious, political, moral, etc.). In his search for authority, the adolescent submits to one or more ideologies because of his internal superego deficiencies, which are inadequately buttressed by the Other. The adolescent gives his allegiance to an apparatus of belief that includes profound involvement in a group or institution. He then becomes dependent on the quality of this environment.

The functioning of the reference object differs according to whether it is a parental object, an object outside the family, involving confrontation and dialogue, or just a neutral ideology (or ideologies). The adolescent's sometimes extreme craving for references may have contrasting results: he may prove unable to find continuity and to work through the novelty of adolescence and collapse into depression or pubertal psychosis; or he may become frozen in conformism due to ideological or superego rigidity.

Conclusion

The sources of genitality, the theory of which is based on the complementarity of the sexes, are symbolized by the pubertal scene. This scene undergoes an elaboration that negotiates with the infantile to reconstruct the subject. The psychic work concerned is moderated by the psychic third-party function, which is always buttressed by a parental transference object.

Any disharmony between the three groups of processes (the pubertal, genital identity, and the referential system) betokens a form of adolescent pathology characteristic of puberty. It disrupts development, preventing the adolescent crisis by rejection of the changes of puberty. The body, as the witness of puberty, becomes the accused.

The adolescent process of becoming-a-subject that accompanies the waning of puberty does not as such define an age of adolescence, which is a sociocultural entity, but is prolonged until the ideal agencies—in particular, the superego—have resumed their (unconscious) autonomy of functioning. Adolescence is an uncertainty or mobility in the process of becoming-a-subject that may give rise to pathology. Its end marks the end of the capacity to change objects. The adult retains a potential for innovation in so far as the processes of adolescence still function unconsciously.

CHAPTER NINE

The process of becoming-a-subject[1] in adolescence

Raymond Cahn

Our view of adolescence today has changed. The individual's history and background are still the determining factors, as illustrated by the model of *Nachträglichkeit*[2]. However, the clinical experience of the last few decades, together with new ideas on causality, casts doubt on the old strictly deterministic approach. That conception has now expanded into a probabilistic vision in which a margin of indeterminacy always persists, in particular in far-from-equilibrium problem situations,

[1][*Translator's note*: The phrase "becoming-a-subject" renders the French word *subjectivation*, a neologism used in particular by the present author, by Philippe Gutton, and by René Roussillon. The process of becoming-a-subject is concerned with differentiation rather than individuation and involves the subjective appropriation of psychic reality. Its exact meaning will become clear from the text of this chapter. I am indebted to Christoph Hering, of Geneva, for suggesting this English translation of *subjectivation*.]

[2][*Translator's note*: This is the word originally used by Freud and translated by Strachey as "deferred action"—a rendering that is now considered controversial because, unlike the French equivalent *après-coup*, it does not give sufficient weight to the idea of retroactive revision.]

so that much greater importance is attached to the random and to the effect of current events. It is therefore appropriate for us to think of psychic functioning in terms not only of its predeterminations and structural constraints, but also of the unforeseen contributions—the noise—of internal and external excitations. These are constantly modifying, calling into question, or conversely fixing and consolidating the psyche's productions and acts through the dialectic of permanence and change, through the possibility of bifurcations and transformations or, conversely, of infinite repetition of the same. Admittedly, the initially infinite and unpredictable virtualities are gradually reduced as the psyche becomes more structured, giving way to increasingly organized forms. But there remains even then a space open to interrogation, to the calling into question of the familiar and the already known, and hence to the possibility of transformation and self-creation. In adolescence, the equilibrium between the two poles of "inside" and "outside" is particularly unstable owing to the imperatives of the pleasure–unpleasure principle. This means that aspirations concerning the object, whether nostalgic or new, may either be kept available or, instead, be excluded; that identity may be confronted, enriched or, alternatively, called into question; and, more generally, that the preconscious and conscious space may be used to the full or, conversely, disabled to a greater or lesser extent (Cahn, 1996).

In view of this twofold perspective, both synchronic and diachronic, all these phenomena taken together may be regarded as a progressive process of becoming-a-subject. This continues from birth until death; while crucially important in the early years of life, it is equally so in adolescence, which is a time of transformation and provisional conclusion, represented through identity-related anxieties and the simultaneously hyper-exciting and hyper-threatening quality of the object. Owing to the extent and intensity of the resulting unbinding activity, much is at stake: will the outcome be a return to the old links or will new ones be created? Particular importance will attach to the existence or otherwise of a margin for indeterminacy in deciding whether the individual remains open to the unknown and the new or persists in the mechanical and the identical. It is at this point that the new constraint—both internal (from the drives) and external (from the environment and from objects)—will ratify, consolidate, call into question, or more or less radically modify the prior forms of the process of becoming-a-subject. This process is one of differentiation rather than of individuation–separation. On the basis of the subject's internal demand for a thought capacity of his own, it allows the appropriation of the sexually mature male or female body and the use of his creativity for disengagement, or disalienation, from the power of the other or from the exercise of that power—thereby transforming the superego and constituting the ego ideal. This process of becoming-a-subject will continue throughout life, and the subject will have to invent himself constantly through the necessary links he has to create as well as in the way those relevant links are perpetually called into question, and in the potential for undoing and remaking them, whether they are the same or different ones, and whether in the same way or differently. I therefore suggest the inclusion in metapsychology of a "subject function" concerned with the various factors implicated in the subjective appropriation of psychic reality. The process of becoming-a-subject, while essentially having to do with the ego, in fact involves all the agencies. At id level, it seems that, contrary to Freud's view, energy circulation is not "free", but that a part of unconscious psychic life is indeed bound. Winnicott, as we know, considered that the drive has an organizing or disorganizing effect according to whether or not it has been integrated in the self. As for the superego, every nuance may be observed between invasive or even destructuring cruelty and ferocity on the one hand and, on the other, its post-oedipal dimension, which has organizing tendencies owing to the anonymity it has acquired and to its protective function. Similarly, we observe at ego level the contrasting elements of alienating identificatory intrusions and structure-promoting identifications, which, while admittedly modelled on the object, in fact originate from the subject. This conception of the subject therefore implies *a certain manner*[3] *of being* and hence the more specific dimension of

[3]The word "manner" comes from the Latin *manuarius*, meaning "of the hand" or "in hand", or, more specifically, of the subject and his capacity to handle in his own way the dough of the world and of the object.

what constitutes the subject, through the requirement of containing, organizing, and conferring meaning upon the constant internal and external changes that affect it. As a result of these changes the subject will become other while remaining to the same extent himself. Such a "manner of being" is alive and creative, even if the subject is overcome by his task, caught up in duplicity and a degree of guilt, incorrigibly megalomanic, separated from an essential or not so essential part of himself, and more or less irremediably exiled from the primary object. It is at this point that analysis can relieve the superego's pressure on, and allow the id greater access to, the ego, thus offering the subject a more open window onto himself and onto the world. That subject will always have been there, underlying and consubstantial with the analytic process and the associated psychic work. Sometimes, however, it will be an absent or insufficient subject, which nevertheless reveals itself to whoever takes it upon himself to seek it out among the range of stratagems to which the psyche is compelled to resort in order to conceal its asphyxiation or alienation. In this case, the psychoanalyst's skill will consist precisely in his ability to identify it behind these masks.

Whereas it is surely a heuristic necessity to make a black-and-white distinction of this kind between capacity and incapacity for becoming-a-subject, in the clinical situation we observe an enormously wide range of individual variations in the degree of this capacity and the forms it assumes, both diachronically and synchronically. Adolescence is thus of crucial importance in the process of becoming-a-subject, which is so extensive in its ramifications that only some of its most significant aspects can be discussed here. After all, it is in adolescence that the internal and external obstacles to the subject's appropriation of his own thoughts, wishes, and identity are reinforced, and that the constant labour of binding and unbinding in all fields, both narcissistic and object-related, is jeopardized by an excess of unbinding. The individual is therefore just as likely to resort to narcissistic regression, frantic externalization, splitting, borrowed identifications, and the desperate search for an authenticity that cannot be found. Whether the disturbance is trivial or serious, at this age the impression gained is of a late revival of depressive and separation anxieties, amplified by the confrontation with the oedipal conflict and the resulting narcissistic wounds, and of a consequent resurgence of early anxieties, hitherto seemingly overcome to a greater or lesser extent. Archaic mechanisms are then mobilized retroactively and assume crucial significance (Cahn, 1991b).

Hence it is understandable that all the many and various unstable and temporary defences deployed by the adolescent to ward off the danger of acquiring the status of a subject persist and become fixed in borderline states when this danger, whatever its origin, ensconces itself in the heart of his being. It may therefore be appropriate to regard these states as being located on the *boundary not between neurosis and psychosis but between the capacity and the incapacity for acceding to subjecthood.* It is as if the psyche had become the prisoner of hostile or hyper-exciting introjects that have henceforth taken up residence in the centre of its being. The basic conflict-avoidance mechanisms of decathexis, splitting, and disavowal to a greater or lesser extent curtail the individual's ability to be the subject of his own conflicts. The same applies when tensions are ejected from the psyche by enactment, projective identification, or even dreams and fantasies. Such incompetence of the protective shield against stimuli, at both narcissistic and object level, seems to be connected with either an excess or a lack of absence on the part of the object between birth and the end of development, which has far-reaching consequences in regard to the very possibility of becoming-a-subject. Indeed, the mastery of the subject by the object seems to be as unrecognized as it is decisive. The same is true of the resulting confusion as to limits and self–other differentiation in all registers subject to the object's influence: identifications at ego, superego, or ego-ideal level, or the space—or lack of space—left to the psyche for a minimum of distancing, self-observation, and self-questioning. The work of Laufer may seem remote from this viewpoint, but his contributions do emphasize the crucial dimension of the developmental breakdown in adolescence, and he therefore maintains that the entire treatment should be directed towards the transference "breakdown" rather than towards the transference "neurosis". What happens is that the deadlocked development so invasively and painfully felt by the adolescent in the here and now is transposed into the unconscious relationship with the therapist. Instead of linking this breakdown to the fantasies and events of early infancy, which the adolescent feels are irrelevant to him except when he uses them for the purposes of defensive idealization, Laufer turns it into a unique instrument in the analytic process. As he points out, "a characteristic of the behaviour of very disturbed adolescents is to express thoughts through action, *with the unconscious need also not to find words or meaning to their actions*" (Laufer, 1996 [my emphasis]). Is this a particularly powerful defence, or is it an inability—absolute or relative—to undertake the work of assigning meaning that is the final stage of the process of becoming-a-subject? If the latter, this would tend to support our view that the relevant pathologies are more than—or indeed different from—an oedipal conflict that the individual is unable to own. We should then certainly be observing the consequences of unbinding activity detrimental not only to the relation to the object but also to the very modalities of mental functioning—that is to say, a disharmony according to the strict dictionary definition: *dis-* = "absence of" and *harmony* = "combination into a consistent whole"[4] (in this case, the whole represented by psychic functioning). This "absence" of a "consistent whole", or *dis*harmony of psychic functioning, is precisely what is at issue in adolescence or post-adolescence. Other concomitant factors involved to varying degrees are the capacity for cathexis and countercathexis (as well as the risks of decathexis), and the balance between the poles of narcissism and the relation to the object. The extreme situations are pathology of narcissistic identification on the one hand and a view of the object as hyper-erotized or hyper-dangerous on the other. Last but not least, the constraints of the drives and those of the object may merge and become telescoped. All these factors may overwhelm the psyche's capacity for work—especially the processes of thought and symbolization—and thus compel the psyche to resort to extreme defences, whose various effects are observed during adolescent analyses in what I shall call a *transference disharmoniosis*. This reflects the forms of psychic dysfunction connected with the obstacles to, or the inability to undertake, the process of becoming-a-subject through the gradual harmonization of its components—for example, in narcissistic pathologies of

---

[4][Translator's note: These definitions are taken from *Webster's Third New International Dictionary*.]

whatever form, which are so organized precisely in order to avoid the dangerous demands of the drives and the equally dangerous encounter with the other. Every introjection and identification is rejected because it is experienced as a penetration inside the subject's boundaries; this position is also a device for systematic evasion of the oedipal situation (Grunberger, 1971). Here, although the process of becoming-a-subject is incomplete, some form of transference may nevertheless be used to facilitate it, through interpretation of the grandiose self and of the rage and devaluation entailed by acknowledgement of the analyst's otherness (Kernberg, 1984; Kohut, 1971). Such a technique will prove futile when the problem is not the incompleteness of the process of becoming-a-subject but a more or less deep-rooted disorder of the very capacity to engage in that process. The constraints imposed on the psyche by the twofold threat of seduction by the drive and mastery by the object then combine or become telescoped, sometimes to the point of preventing the ego from undertaking this task of disalienation by itself, although this is the only possible way of genuinely elucidating and disengaging from the transference situation, a process that is itself moulded by the subject's primitive relations. The result is a fusion of the analyst with the internal object, of the analyst with the setting, or even of the analysis with life, while the "as if" dimension that ought to underlie the working-through of the transference appears to a greater or lesser extent to vanish or to get lost. In my view, we are here on the boundary between the capacity and the incapacity to undertake the process of becoming-a-subject, so that the analyst himself has to be the agent of that process when necessary.

This situation, in which the psyche is no longer the locus only of productions to be integrated but also of a radical otherness implanted in its very heart by the object, is seen on an even more massive scale in adolescent psychotic breakdown, whether or not reversible. The model is that of Tausk's patient, in whom the disruptive, persecutory character of genital sexuality, projected into the delusional theme of the influencing machine ("I am sexuality"), is indicative of a primary narcissistic fault (Tausk, 1919). This overdetermination is observed at three levels in adolescent psychotics: (1) a confusion of identificatory reference points; (2) permeation by both internal and external sexual excitation, which they desperately try to bind in a wide variety of ways; and (3) a primary object that seeks to preserve primitive non-distinction instead of favouring progressive differentiation, in a situation of alienating mastery or of indefinite excitation connected with the object's shortcomings. What is then lacking is the external protective shield against stimuli that is essential for binding and organizing the internal and external excitations in a structuring autoerotism that differentiates between inside and outside—i.e. the basic outline of a self and subsequently of the subject. Such a shield would, by internalization of the maternal function of warding off stimuli, allow the gradual differentiation of subject and object and the binding of affects to the object in representations and symbols—which is the fundamental condition for primary repression and the possibility of structuring identifications.

A threat of this kind to the narcissistic foundations and to the relation to the object is observed in adolescence in all kinds of circumstances. A particular example is when the individual attempts to respond as an autonomous subject with a sexual identity of his own to a family environment determined at all costs to maintain its mastery over him or to reject him while disavowing the fact. Another is when the subject himself needs the permanent presence of the external object as the only possible reassurance against invasion by excess excitation. The result will be a psychotogenic collusion between a present-day identity conflict and early narcissistic fragility, which is all the more formidable when accompanied by parental lies, secrets, or double binds. These may concern the origin of the subject, his place in the sequence of generations, or his own or his parents' experiences concerning himself, so that he finds himself under the sway of the other's words and deeds, with "secondary violence"—covert or manifest rejection—taking over from the early violence and rejection (Aulagnier, 1975).

The role of this *cumulative unbinding* is thus clearly very important, and there is every indication that it has taken place on a massive scale in the early years of life. During childhood, the subject is then left totally at the mercy of the object, so that he silently falls victim to the yoke of rigidity, conformism, inhibition, and poverty of cathexes—apart from some transient erratic explosions—until the post-pubertal breakdown. Both in the way it flares up and in its insidious, devastating manifestations when the Oedipus complex is reactivated in adolescence, this breakdown amplifies to an intolerable pitch the truly incestuous or murderous character of the interrelationships within such a triangle. Whereas the Oedipus complex does indeed prove to be the central organizer in adolescence, the catastrophe of psychosis is not to be attributed to its failure. Such a breakdown implies an organization that prevents the subject from owning the oedipal situation and turns it into a psychic brick wall. Which strictly psychotic defences are in fact deployed will depend on the specific distance from such an experience or its actual occurrence. The phenomena concerned are principally *the various forms of failure to take account of internal and external reality*, with the associated splitting, extending from disavowal to greater or lesser degrees of decathexis and—depending on the intensity and forms of the process—culminating in various mechanisms such as delusion, hallucination, and the like. These mechanisms take over more or less for "their own account" the tangled skein made up of the subject's own and others' psychic productions, and the subject finds himself so to speak excluded to a greater or lesser extent from the ego's consequent reconstructions.

Our therapeutic options—situated beyond the most clamorous symptomatic manifestations—attempt to bypass the problems of disavowal and splitting and to gain access to this primitive fault by the offer of a containing setting that will afford protection against stimuli. This setting must guarantee adequate continuity, be based on an essentially paternal law, and make available a transitional space or play area within which a kind of primary symbolization might be possible, sheltered from anything that might remotely or otherwise suggest mastery or violence on the part of the object. The repetition compulsion will, of course, disturb or compromise this aim, so that the primitive fault, as well as the transgenerational burden, may be actualized in complex and troublesome fashion in the transference and countertransference. It may then be possible for the "therapist–object" for the first time to offer the subject other experiences, on the basis of which his narcissistic foundations will be consolidated and the level of excitation will be reduced, so that he need no longer resort to such disabling defences (Cahn, 1991a).

In this case, unlike the neurotic situation, where it is necessary to consider only the internal objects within a basically reliable and silent setting, *the setting itself proves to be the object of the process*. This is the only possible genuinely psychoanalytic approach to tackling, other than *in absentia aut in effigie*, the decisive impact of the external object and the environment in these typical cases. Meaning can be assigned anew to the many forms of expression of the repetition compulsion that seemingly or actually lack meaning or whose meaning has been stripped away. The healing techniques of so-called primitive societies are not dissimilar from our psychotherapeutic approach. In both cases the aim is *to grasp as tightly as possible what seem to us to be the most specifically psychotic aspects—or, rather, those that tend to deprive the individual of his subjecthood—of the disorders with which we are concerned*. However, unlike Lévi-Strauss, we consider that words, while truly acknowledging the subject's ills or affliction and giving him back a system of understanding that is both personal and universally shared, *cannot have any effect whatsoever unless rooted both in affect and in narcissistic identification with the other*. The same mechanism is also observed in the undoing of the mastery to which anyone who looks after or treats psychotics is subjected, where the essential point is to recognize what is thereby being mutually experienced, i.e. *what had thus been experienced but never mentally assimilated by any of the protagonists*. It will then be possible to formulate this in the group's common area of illusion or to offer a non-alienating response in the subject–object relationship.

In our adolescents, whatever responses the ego has been compelled to adopt (borderline states or miscellaneous psychotic organizations), the outcome will depend on whether or not space is left for an attempt at detachment, by the making of new links, from the compulsive repetition of the unbearable, which the psychotic defences seek at such high cost to confront.

The approach proposed here, however imperfect, attempts to take overall account of the situation arising when psychotic manifestations, whether limited or invasive, appear in adolescence. Every adolescent's conquest and appropriation of self and world are surely mediated by the appropriation of his own body, and always on the basis of the relevant organizations laid down by mental processes at the beginning of life. Now this appropriation—not only of the subject's body but also of his position as a sexually mature male or female individual in the sequence of generations—necessarily entails conflict and contradiction and calls for passage *through a prior phase—whether virtual or, as is usually the case, concretely experienced—of anxious questioning about what was familiar but has now suddenly become uncanny, and of deprivation of the body and of the world.*

This is the point at which the risk of dispossession arises. If this dispossession proves intolerable to the subject, he will either have to go to the lengths of self-exclusion or self-decathexis or be compelled to see it as possession. Here, too, the fate of the area of illusion is determined. Depending on the quality and power of both the internal object and the external object, this area will allow the subject to express his own truth and view of the world—or alternatively it may lure him into a closed ideology or delusion, alienating or imprisoning him and distorting his world. Another possibility is that, panic-stricken when all is thereby called into question again or even unable to conceive this situation, he may remain inside this timeless time, abandoning his psyche and body to the other, devoid of thoughts or wishes of his own, an automaton at the mercy of the other's omnipotence. When this calling-into-question eventually falls due, as it inevitably will, the outcome will be determined by the subject's capacity for binding, autonomy, and symbolization, or, conversely, by the disabling of this capacity. This is the moment of truth as to the actual and/or assigned role of the object in terms of its provision or non-provision of the psychic space in which the subject can live a psychic life of his own, with his own conflicts, in a world experienced as real. This concept of the process of becoming-a-subject, as currently envisaged by many authors (Balier, 1997; Birraux, 1994; Gutton, 1996; Roussillon, 1995), combines the radical selfhood of the psyche and the absolute necessity of the other, the constraints of the drives and those of the object. It throws new light on adolescent psychopathology, which should be seen as the non-completion of the concluding phase of this process.

CHAPTER TEN

Normality and pathology in adolescence

François Ladame and Maja Perret-Catipovic

The question of normality and pathology in adolescence has always been controversial and remains so. The issue is not discussed in detail in this chapter, which is not intended as a substitute for a treatise on psychopathology. We confine ourselves to laying down some markers to facilitate the understanding of normal and abnormal developments and to putting forward some essential criteria for appraisal of the main characteristics of psychic functioning. The initial taking of bearings discussed here, which falls short of a detailed assessment calling for specific training, is necessary if not sufficient, because it already has far-reaching implications for the adolescent's future.

In the wake of Winnicott (1961), many still play down the most violent tokens of mental anguish, such as suicide attempts, and advocate a minimum of therapeutic intervention or even none at all. Whereas this trivialization of adolescent disorders certainly occurs, the opposite may also be the case, when all conflictual and disturbing manifestations of adolescence are seen as pathological.

One way of avoiding these twin perils would be to postulate that the meaning of adolescent subjects' manifestations and symptoms not only differs from that which might be assigned to their counterparts in children or adults, but is also specific to the process of development. *There is no adolescence without a crisis of adolescence.* The crisis bears witness to a critical phase of human development and is at the same time the expression of psychic work undertaken in the service of that development. However, it does not follow that anything and everything (for example, all the known manifestations of psychopathology) can be subsumed within this concept, as was for many years the case. The unfortunate consequence of this approach was to prevent diagnosis and the recommendation of therapy for young people. Today, we are well aware of the deterioration of patients with manifest psychic disorders in adolescence, who did not receive proper treatment on the grounds that they were undergoing an "adolescent crisis".

In its etymological sense of a moment of "decision" [*krisis*], the adolescent crisis is indeed the inescapable time of life that leads on to adult sexuality. Defined in this way, however, it covers only the normal process. On the basis of clinical observation and follow-up studies, interest has gradually come to focus, not so much on the crisis phenomenon as such as on the *outcome of the crisis*, which may be variable.

In outline, the crisis accompanying the period of pubertal transformations culminates, in favourable cases, in a higher level of organization and psychic functioning than before. This gain is reflected, in particular, in greater autonomy with respect to the outside world and better self–other differentiation. The unfavourable outcome, betokening the onset of pathology and its retinue of associated symptoms, is a regression to modes of functioning inferior to the pre-crisis forms. Between these two extremes may lie an intermediate position that is by definition unstable: a kind of endless crisis state in which both progression and regression beckon but each of these paths is blocked by an insurmountable barrier.

Some major psychic disorders of adolescent onset appear like a bolt from the blue and inevitably raise the *question of continuity or discontinuity with childhood disorders*. A less black-and-white approach to this still topical issue is surely appropriate. Some of the most severe disorders manifest in childhood will continue in adolescence with modifications due to the reality of the changes of puberty, whereas others give the impression of leapfrogging the new reality and developing out of time. What of the severe disorders that emerge only at the time of adolescence? The constructions and reconstructions possible in a therapeutic setting usually show that these major breakdowns occur in subjects who have been unable to produce a genuine infantile neurosis—that is, a framing structure whereby the threats to narcissism can be referred to castration anxiety rather than catastrophic anxiety. By a framing structure, we mean also the constitution of a psychic container (Bion, 1962) or the setting up of a "protective shield against stimuli for the inside" (Ladame, 1991), which will prove its worth precisely at the time of the crisis of adolescence. The inevitable bursting asunder of the infantile topographical organization will remain contained, so that its fragments are not scattered to the winds with concomitant loss by the self of the self. It would thus clearly be a hazardous venture to "predict" the form a childhood disorder might assume after puberty, because it is virtually impossible to determine in advance how continuity and discontinuity will then be intermixed. One of the parameters of normal development is the preservation of the dialectical link between these two opposites.

A possible interpretation of this "bolt from the blue" is offered in this chapter.

The crisis and its outcomes

Let us review the situation from the beginning. The reality principle governing the prepubertal child's psychic life is that of his actual physical and psychosexual limitations; this is a *de facto* impotence concomitant with the omnipotence of thought that protects narcissism. The child's body is separate from that of his parents, but he is incapable of fulfilling his sexual role in material reality. The content of the identifications implies a position of incapacity relative to the parental imagos, so that the initial situation is as shown below (FIGURE 1).

A twofold seesaw movement is wrought by puberty (FIGURE 2): bodily impotence turns into bodily potency in the orgasmic and procreative sense; and the omnipotence of thought gives way to the acknowledgement of finitude, with its implications of the universality of death, the difference between the sexes, and the

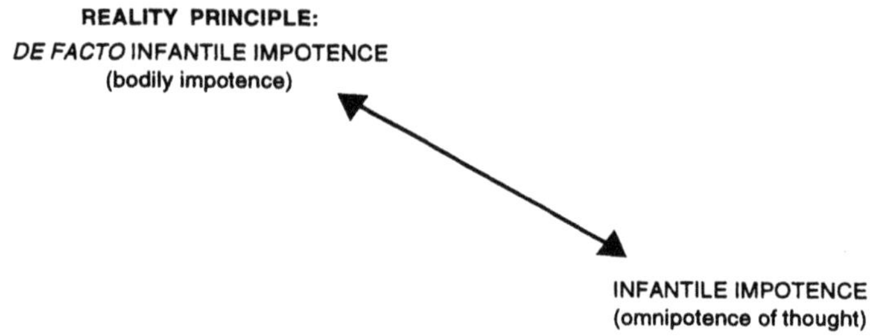

FIGURE 1. Before puberty

difference between the generations. The movement's fulcrum is the change in the reality principle.

The body, of course, lies at the heart of the question of adolescent development. Loss of the illusions of perfection and bisexuality is a precondition for the possibility of cathecting the body of a man or woman, which is a diktat of puberty. Now our relationship with reality depends on our relationship with our bodies. Sensory impressions and lived experience are filtered by

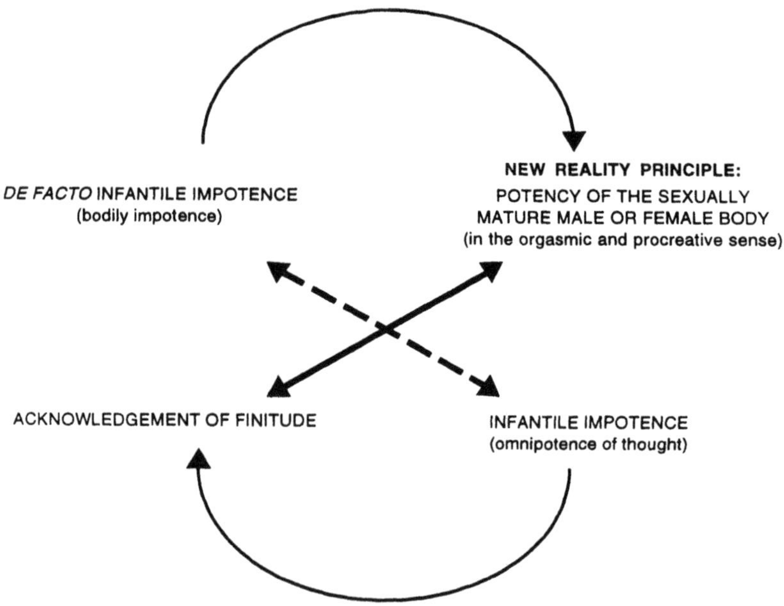

FIGURE 2. From puberty

the body, which decisively shapes the representation we make of the outside world. The body thus being the interface between inside and outside, the quality of its narcissistic cathexis after puberty will self-evidently determine the way in which the outside world is apprehended. In other words, if the body is cathected with a mainly negative narcissistic quality, external reality will be experienced as persecutory.

We have just referred to the representation that we make for ourselves of the outside world. A function whereby representation can be distinguished from perception is also needed. That function is *reality testing*. According to Freud, reality testing enables us to distinguish between, on the one hand, what is not real, what is only within, what is confined to a representation, and, on the other, what is real—that is, what also exists outside (Freud, 1917d, 1925h). He tells us, too, that loss is a precondition for the establishment of reality testing: "objects shall have been lost which once brought real satisfaction" (Freud, 1925h, p. 238). Here a difficulty arises. There has certainly been an object that afforded satisfaction on the level of need (self-preservation), but what might that object have been in the field of sexuality? Only autoerotism, coupled with the omnipotence of thought, permits narcissistic "survival" in the face of the affront of infantile impotence.

We are reminded in *Beyond the Pleasure Principle* (Freud, 1920g, p. 20) that infantile experiences were primarily sources of unpleasure. The extinction of the "early efflorescence of infantile sexual life" takes place in the worst circumstances and leaves behind the bitter taste of failure. So does our difficulty not border upon an aporia? And does it not condemn reality testing to remain for all time somewhat rickety in the field of sexuality—that is, to maintain a vagueness, an absence of clear boundaries, around this object: is it an object to be found or in fact one to be re-found? This brings us to one of the paradoxes of adolescence, because development specifically involves the body, sexuality, and reality testing, and because the latter must be the guarantor of boundaries—in particular, those between inside and outside. At the same time, however, although this paradox—or aporia, if it be such—complicates our human lives, it greatly mitigates the apparent rigidity of the distinction between normality and pathology; this fact can surely only be welcomed.

Let us return to the question of what is to be (re)found and of this hypothetical object of satisfaction. Infantile sexuality bears the stamp of inferiority, impotence, and the tragic (Freud, 1920g). It is narcissistically bearable only through the promise inherent in it. If it were a matter of "re-finding" something, what is re-found would be the horror of this impotence. Yet for many it seems difficult if not impossible to give up this unsatisfying past and to work through its loss. Why should this be? The prepubertal child's "revolt" against his real physical and psychosexual limitations determines the direction of the whole of psychic functioning by way of the omnipotence of thought, which promises better days in the future ("when I grow up, . . ."). Now, just at the time when the incestuous wishes could be fulfilled (orgasmic and procreative potency having been fully acquired), they must be renounced precisely because incest and parricide have become possible. This renunciation is a demand both of the superego and of civilization. What substitutive promise would be sufficiently attractive to make one wish to carry on regardless, if not the hope of freeing oneself from repetition?

How then can we do without a conceptualization of adolescence centred on its innovative and revolutionary aspects, which alone can enable the subject to emerge from repetition? The elation of adolescence might be partly due to the dimly glimpsed possibility of freedom at last from the infantile triad of impotence, inferiority, and the tragic. The terror would be of excessive uncertainty about being able to escape this fate.

The question of incest and parricide, too, calls for an answer, because these wishes cannot be "lost" (Freud, 1900a). This answer necessarily involves recourse to repression and to the preconscious—that is, to a compromise or artifice: as far as his superego is concerned, the subject renounces his oedipal wishes, while allowing them to persist in the unconscious. In order to be satisfying in economic terms, this also entails a shift from autoerotism to the search for an object. Autoerotic satisfaction is blocked in so far as the subject can no longer conceal from himself the fact that the narcissistic object of satisfaction is also the incestuous object.

In the *pathological situation*, the twofold seesaw movement is prevented (FIGURE 3), the main obstacle being the difficulty, or even impossibility, of giving up infantile omnipotence and/or the re-

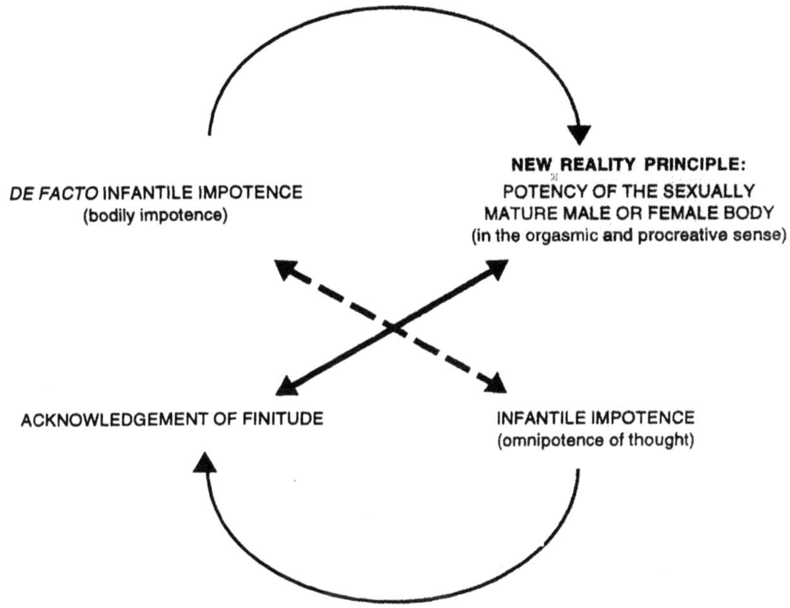

FIGURE 3. Pathological solution

fusal to give it up. However, assumption of the sexually mature male or female adult body cannot be reconciled with the preservation of infantile omnipotence, because the combination would mean that incest and parricide had been consummated. The only possible solution remaining in this case is *splitting of the ego*[1] and disavowal.

---

[1]This is the term used by Freud (1940e [1938]) to denote the coexistence within the ego of two opposing attitudes towards external reality. These two attitudes exist side by side without mutually influencing each other—that is, without the formation of a dialectical link between them. Splitting goes hand-in-hand with disavowal, the prototype of which is the disavowal of castration. This model must be clearly distinguished from that of repression and the return of the repressed and is essential for an understanding of the severe pathologies of adolescence, such as, in particular, those covered by the concepts of deadlock and developmental breakdown (Laufer & Laufer, 1984).

The split is a reaction by the ego to the trauma inherent in the necessity and simultaneous impossibility of the twofold seesaw movement. In one part of the ego, incest and parricide have "happened" and omnipotent narcissism is "avenged", whereas the other part of the ego is under the sway of disavowal of the drama that has been consummated and functions under the illusion of angelism; it finds itself compelled either not to cathect the male or female body or to cathect it as responsible for badness, making it a target of hate. This "solution" might appear tempting were it not fraudulent: infantile omnipotence is preserved at the cost of the impossibility of becoming-a-subject (see Cahn, Chapter 9 of this book). The division of the subject constitutes an anti-narcissistic solution, because it introduces a non-cohesion of the ego and an absence of continuity in the sense of being.

A final solution to the problem of incest is also necessary for the construction of the categories of past, present, and future. When incest is confined within the unconscious, it is manifested solely in returns of the repressed and in dreams. Conversely, when the incestuous pressure is too strong, the "timelessness" of incest prevails over linear temporality. Again, owing to the fact of narcissistic fragility, the search for the object is stamped with the threat it presents to the ego. On this level, too, the subject finds himself deadlocked: what is most sought after and possibly desired, or indeed most indispensable to ontological "survival", is what constitutes the greatest danger for the individual. On the level of sexuality, the subject's inescapable dependence, for the satisfaction of his own desire, on the other and on the other's desire becomes a source of panic anxiety and possibly of phobic mechanisms; on the more general level of object relations, it becomes necessary to find compromises between dependence and self-sufficiency that are by definition wanting. In the limit, the outcome will be a relation to a part-object which is denied its capacity to desire—a relation to an object over which control and mastery can be exerted.

Another consequence of the absence of a dialectical link between the split-off parts of the ego is the non-existence of psychic conflictuality and of work to seek compromise solutions. This situation will have cognitive repercussions. The adolescents concerned are often unaware of the contradictions that they express in their words and lives, and, what is more, are incapable of doing anything about them. In so far as psychic conflictuality is the engine of development, that development cannot continue in adolescence if it is absent. This contributes to deadlock or foreclosure, to use the terminology of Laufer & Laufer (1984).

The split that, as we have just shown, served to maintain an illusion of omnipotence also has a more adaptive function: it preserves a topographical organization, albeit mutilated, and prevents the collapse of that organization. It would be wrong to see the absence of a topography characteristic of pathology, on the one hand, and its presence as the token of normality, on the other, as antitheses. The inescapable phenomenon of the "pubertal" (Gutton, 1991) is like an explosion, which is followed by a process of repair, with the formation of healing scar tissue, whereby the same topography is innovatively reorganized. What is characteristic of pathology is the impossibility of re-repressing the pubertal scenes, which are by nature crude, cruel, and consequently disorganizing. The issue here is the functionality of the preconscious. Depending on its quality, trauma-like topographical subsidences (for example, moments of raptus or of breakdown) may occur in the ongoing process. These are necessarily followed by a reorganization. Unlike the potential in the normal situation, the reorganization here is to a regressive, pathological level, at the expense of the progressive differentiation that is characteristic of development.

In our view, at present the best way to conceptualize what the subject experiences—and at the same time does not experience, because he is both there and not there—is in terms of trauma. Owing to the temporary obliteration of the ego (proper to the trauma situation) and, by extension, the temporary obliteration of topography, what is experienced fails to be registered clearly as either representation or perception. In this connection we must again emphasize the role of the preconscious in its functions of binding, unbinding, and rebinding. A functioning preconscious allows what has been unbound to be contained, so that free energy can be displaced and re-bound.

Some criteria for assessing adolescent psychic functioning

Assessment in adolescence always relates to a *process*—namely, the one whereby a fixed and irreversible sexual identity is established with adulthood. The consistent thread running through this process will therefore be the vicissitudes of the narcissistic cathexis of the sexually mature male or female body. The reference to the developmental process indicates the specificity of the assessment of psychic functioning in the adolescent as compared with the adult, even if most of the criteria reviewed here also apply to other ages. On completion of his assessment, the clinician must be able to answer the following questions: What stage of development has this young man—or woman—reached? Is the process of development still under way, or is it deadlocked or even threatened with foreclosure?

Similarly, *reality testing* cannot and must not be seen in simple binary terms as being either present or absent. We need to know how far the adolescent can "adapt" to the inevitable instability of reality testing in the field of sexuality without thereby forfeiting his sexual life, capacity for daydreaming, and link with reality. The most difficult assessments are those in which the picture is dominated by inhibition. Even an experienced clinician may find it hard to decide whether and to what extent this might still be defensive. Inhibition (of mental activity) may be a way of "adapting" to the difficulty mentioned above, by putting a stop to daydreams, thought, and wishes (as well as, sometimes, the body). Unfortunately, however, seemingly identical clinical pictures may merely be masks for a void when the activity of thought has been destroyed.

As to the *topographical organization*, the assessment must focus on the functionality of the *preconscious*. This is best appreciated through daydreaming activity, which indicates flexibility in the interplay of repression and the return of the repressed. Paradoxically, the subject must also be capable of enduring those moments of dysfunction of the preconscious agency when the "uncanny" comes to the fore. The more it is possible for functionality to coexist with moments of dysfunction, the less problematical the adolescent process will be. These moments are connected with the vacillation of reality testing, with impressions of *déjà vu* and of earlier experience repeated, which, according to Freud (1919h), have to do with fantasies of returning to the womb and hence of the fulfilment of incest. Such "uncanny" moments signify that the incestuous and parricidal wishes are no longer confined to the unconscious, and that they are temporarily intruding into consciousness without being disguised by the preconscious. They reflect an ongoing labour of refunctionalization of the preconscious.

With regard to the *ego functions*, particular attention must be devoted to the interplay of progression and regression. As Blos (1967) points out, regression is not in itself pathological. Conversely, a problem *is* presented by the impossibility of maintaining dialectical tension between these opposites and hence of associating the regressive movement with one of evolution, whether this impossibility is reflected in exclusive recourse to regression or in an incapacity to yield to it temporarily. Regression may be either normal or pathological and is not a criterion for differential diagnosis. Among the defence mechanisms, it is important to distinguish between those with and those without ego-mutilating effects. Splitting, disavowal, and massive projective identification are mutilating, whereas the defences deployed to mitigate the disruptiveness of energy cathexes (repression, displacement, and isolation) are more in the service of the ego. Projection, the mechanism that reigns supreme in adolescence, is no indicator of normality or pathology.

It is important, too, to assess the capacity for tolerating *frustration*. Tolerating frustration means toleration of the fact that the affront of infantile sexual impotence can never be avenged. The more an adolescent is assailed by these problems and by ideas of "vengeance", the less tolerant he will be of frustration, a situation that will be reflected principally by short-circuits in thought.

Attention must also be paid to the capacity to preserve a *link between libido and aggression* as well as *between narcissistic cathexis and object cathexis*. Normally, the subject's wealth of object cathexes reinforces his narcissistic cathexes, while, conversely, a solid narcissistic cathexis allows him to search for the object without feeling threatened (with being swallowed up). All the same, when the young adolescent is harshly confronted with the problems of gains and losses, his embrittled narcissism must be able to call upon a double or *alter ego* for support. In as much as this double can be used transitionally to perform a re-narcissizing function, it may in the same proportion become an obstacle to object-relating, when love of the "same" is deployed at the expense of love of a "different" other. This example again shows how important it is to beware of setting too much store by a single criterion and to make sure that we take account of the developmental process as a whole.

There are, of course, exceptions to this rule. The main exception concerns the act, or more precisely *enactment*, which we distinguish from action (Ladame, 1991). The aim of the drive is action. From this point of view, an adolescent who is incapable of acting should worry us. However, so should an adolescent who is incapable of not acting—that is, one who has lost control of his deeds and gestures (here we prefer the term "enactment"), who presents a great danger to himself and possibly also to others. It is in our view therefore essential to distinguish between "action" and "enactment". The latter term covers all uncontrollable compulsive acts involving the subject himself or the other: running away, theft, violence or suicide attempts, abuse of alcohol, medicines or drugs, gambling, high-risk behaviour, sex, or fasting. Action, by contrast, serves for experimentation to discover the limits of the sexually mature male or female body and to integrate the newly acquired potential of the drives. In this respect an active relationship with the subject's own body is essential: this will involve, in the case of a boy, the capacity to touch the penis and to masturbate, and in girls the choice of clothing and make-up.

To conclude this brief survey, we would emphasize that a major risk when the process of development begins to go wrong (whether clamorously or tacitly) is the adoption of a *perverse solution*. While difficult to assess, it is incumbent upon us to recognize such a tendency owing to its prognostic indications: termination of the process initiated by the pubertal explosion of puberty, but with a pathological outcome; and extinction of anxiety and psychic suffering, but by sleight of hand. Truck with the genital whole object, as the conquest of adolescence (even if accompanied by the inevitable frustration of the confrontation with otherness), is replaced by the use of a part-object, the other, the subject's own body, or a thing, which may be pressed into service in any way he pleases.

REFERENCES

Adatto, C. P. (1958). Ego reintegration observed in analysis of late adolescents. *International Journal of Psycho-Analysis, 39*: 172–177.

Aichhorn, A. (1925). *Wayward Youth.* New York: Viking Press, 1948.

Aristotle. *Rhetorica. The Works of Aristotle, Vol. XI.* Oxford: Clarendon Press, 1946.

Aulagnier, P. (1975). *La violence de l'interprétation.* Paris: Presses Universitaires de France.

Aulagnier, P. (1984). Telle une "zone sinistrée". *Adolescence, 2*: 9–21.

Balier, C. (1997). *Psychanalyse des comportements sexuels violents.* Paris: Presses Universitaires de France.

Bernfeld, S. (1923). Concerning a typical form of male puberty. *Adolescent Psychiatry, 20*: 51–65, 1995.

Bibring, G. L. (1959). Some considerations of the psychological processes in pregnancy. *Psychoanalytic Study of the Child, 14*: 113–121.

Bion, W. (1962). *Learning from Experience.* New York: Basic Books.

Birraux, A. (1994). *Eloge de la phobie.* Paris: Presses Universitaires de France.

Blos, P. (1954). Prolonged adolescence. *American Journal of Orthopsychiatry, 24*: 733–742.

Blos, P. (1962). *On Adolescence. A Psychoanalytic Interpretation.* New York: Free Press of Glencoe.

Blos, P. (1963). The concept of acting out in relation to the adolescent process. *Journal of the American Academy of Child Psychiatry, 2*: 118–143.

Blos, P. (1967). The second individuation process of adolescence. *Psychoanalytic Study of the Child, 22*: 162–186.

Blos, P. (1984). Son and father. *Journal of the American Psychoanalytic Association, 32*: 301–324.

Burlingham, D. (1952). *Twins: A Study of Three Pairs of Identical Twins.* London: Imago; New York: International Universities Press.

Cahn, R. (1991a). *Adolescence et folie. Les déliaisons dangereuses.* Paris: Presses Universitaires de France.

Cahn, R. (1991b). Du sujet. *Revue Française de Psychanalyse, 55*: 1353–1488.

Cahn, R. (1996). L'adolescence en l'an 2'000. *Cahiers de Psychologie Clinique, 6*: 35–44.

Dessoir, M. (1894). Zur Psychologie der Vita sexualis. *Allgemeine Zeitschrift für Psychiatrie und psychisch-gerichtliche Medizin, 50*: 941–975.

Deutsch, H. (1925). *Psychoanalyse der weiblichen Sexualfunktionen.* Vienna: Internationale Psychoanalytische Verlag.

Eissler, K. R. (1950). Ego-psychological implications of the psychoanalytic treatment of delinquents. *Psychoanalytic Study of the Child, 5*: 97–121.

Ellis, H. (1913). *Studies in the Psychology of Sex, Vol. 3.* Philadelphia.

Ellis, H. (1928). *Studies in the Psychology of Sex, Vol. 7.* Philadelphia.

Federn, P. (1952). *Ego Psychology and the Psychoses.* New York: Basic Books. [Reprinted London: Karnac Books, 1977.]

Ferenczi, S. (1924). *Thalassa. A Theory of Genitality.* New York: Psychoanalytic Quarterly, 1938. [Reprinted London: Karnac Books, 1989.]

Fraiberg, S. (1955). Some considerations on the introduction to therapy in puberty. *Psychoanalytic Study of the Child, 10*: 264–286.

Freeman, T., Cameron, J. L., & Mc Ghie, A. (1958). *Chronic Schizophrenia.* London: Tavistock Publications/New York: International Universities Press.

Freud, A. (1936). *The Ego and the Mechanisms of Defense.* New York: International Universities Press, 1946.

Freud, A. (1951). A connection between the states of negativism and of emotional surrender (Hörigkeit). Paper read at the International Psycho-Analytical Congress, Amsterdam, August 1951. Summary in *International Journal of Psycho-Analysis, 33* (1952): 265.

Freud, A. (1952). The mutual influences in the development of Ego and Id: introduction to the discussion. *Psychoanalytic Study of the Child, 7*: 42–50.

Freud, A. (1958). Adolescence. *Psychoanalytic Study of the Child, 13*: 255–278.

Freud, A. (1965). *Normality and Pathology in Childhood*. New York: International Universities Press.

Freud, S. (1895b). On the grounds for detaching a particular syndrome from neurasthenia under the description "anxiety neurosis". *S.E. 3*: 85–115.

Freud, S. (1900a). *The Interpretation of Dreams. S.E. 4–5*: 1–621.

Freud, S. (1904a). Freud's psycho-analytic procedure. *S.E. 7*: 247–254.

Freud, S. (1905c). *Jokes and Their Relation to the Unconscious. S.E. 8*.

Freud, S. (1905d). *Three Essays on the Theory of Sexuality. S.E. 7*: 123–243.

Freud, S. (1906a). My views on the part played by sexuality in the aetiology of the neuroses. *S.E. 7*: 269–279.

Freud, S. (1908e). Creative writers and day-dreaming. *S.E. 9*: 141–153.

Freud, S. (1909c). Family romances. *S.E. 9*: 235–241.

Freud, S. (1909d). Notes upon a case of obsessional neurosis. *S.E. 10*: 151–249.

Freud, S. (1910h). A special type of choice of object made by man (Contributions to the psychology of love I). *S.E. 11*: 163–175.

Freud, S. (1912d). On the universal tendency to debasement in the sphere of love (contributions to the psychology of love II). *S.E. 11*: 177–190.

Freud, S. (1912–1913). *Totem and Taboo. S.E. 13*: 1–161.

Freud, S. (1914c). On narcissism: an introduction. *S.E. 14*: 67–102.

Freud, S. (1916–1917). *Introductory Lectures on Psycho-Analysis. S.E. 15–16*.

Freud, S. (1917d). Metapsychological supplement to the theory of dreams. *S.E. 14*: 217–235.

Freud, S. (1918b). From the history of an infantile neurosis. *S.E. 17*: 1–122.

Freud, S. (1919e). "A child is being beaten". *S.E. 17*: 175–204.

Freud, S. (1919h). The "uncanny". *S.E. 17*: 217–256.

Freud, S. (1920a). The psychogenesis of a case of female homosexuality. *S.E. 18*: 145–172.

Freud, S. (1920g). *Beyond the Pleasure Principle. S.E. 18*: 1–64.

Freud, S. (1923b). *The Ego and the Id. S.E. 19*: 1–59.

Freud, S. (1923e). The infantile genital organization of the libido. *S.E. 19*: 139–145.

Freud, S. (1924c). The economic problem of masochism. *S.E. 19*: 155–170.

Freud, S. (1925h). Negation. *S.E. 19*: 233–239.

Freud, S. (1925j). Some psychological consequences of the anatomical distinction between the sexes. *S.E. 19*: 241–258.

Freud, S. (1926d). *Inhibitions, Symptoms and Anxiety. S.E. 20*: 75–174.

Freud, S. (1930a). *Civilization and Its Discontents. S.E. 21*: 57–145.

Freud, S. (1931b). Female sexuality. *S.E. 21*: 221–243.

Freud, S. (1933a). *New Introductory Lectures on Psycho-Analysis. S.E. 22*: 1–182.

Freud, S. (1937c). Analysis terminable and interminable. *S.E. 23*: 209–253.

Freud, S. (1940e [1938]). Splitting of the Ego in the process of defence. *S.E. 23*: 271–278.

Freud, S. (1950a [1887–1902]). *The Origins of Psychoanalysis, Letters to Wilhelm Fliess, Drafts and Notes 1887–1902*. London: Imago, 1954/ New York: Basic Books, 1954 [partially reprinted in *S.E. 1*: 173–397 (including "A project for a scientific psychology", 1895)].

Friedman, M., Glasser, M., Laufer, E., Laufer, M., & Wohl, M. (1972). Attempted suicide and self-mutilation in adolescence. *International Journal of Psycho-Analysis, 53*: 179–183.

Geleerd, E.R. (1961). Some aspects of ego vicissitudes in adolescence. *Journal of the American Psychoanalytic Association, 9*: 394–405.

Geleerd, E.R. (1964). Adolescence and adaptive regression. *Bulletin of the Menninger Clinic, 28*: 302–308.

Green, A. (1993). *Le travail du négatif*. Paris: Minuit.

Grunberger, B. (1971). *Le narcissisme*. Paris: Payot.

Gutton, P. (1991). *Le pubertaire*. Paris: Presses Universitaires de France.

Gutton, P. (1996). *Adolescens*. Paris: Presses Universitaires de France.

Hartmann, H. (1939). *Ego Psychology and the Problem of Adaptation*. New York: International Universities Press, 1958.

Inhelder, B., & Piaget J. (1958). *The Growth of Logical Thinking from Childhood to Adolescence.* New York: Basic Books.

Jeammet, P. (1980). Réalité interne et réalité externe. *Revue Française de Psychanalyse, 44*: 481–521.

Jeammet, P. (1990). Les destins de l'auto-érotisme à l'adolescence. In: A.-M. Alléon, O. Morvan, & S. Lebovici (Eds.), *Devenir "adulte"* (pp. 52–79). Paris: Presses Universitaires de France.

Jones, E. (1922). Some problems of adolescence. In: *Papers on Psycho-Analysis* (pp. 389–406). London: Baillière, Tindal & Cox, 1948. [Reprinted London: Karnac Books, 1977.]

Katan, M. (1950). Structural aspects of a case of schizophrenia. *Psychoanalytic Study of the Child, 5*: 175–211.

Katan-Angel, A. (1937). The role of displacement in agoraphobia. *International Journal of Psycho-Analysis, 32*: 41–50, 1951.

Kernberg, O. F. (1984). *Severe Personality Disorders. Psychotherapeutic Strategies.* New Haven, CT: Yale University Press.

Kestemberg, E. (1962). L'identité et l'identification chez les adolescents. *Psychiatrie de l'Enfant, 5*: 441–522.

Kestemberg, E. (1980). Notule sur la crise de l'adolescence. De la déception à la conquête. *Revue Française de Psychanalyse, 44*: 523–530.

Klein, M. (1922). Inhibitions and difficulties at puberty. In: *Love, Guilt and Reparation and Other Works 1921–1945. The Writings of Melanie Klein, Vol. 1* (pp. 54–58). London: Hogarth Press, 1981 [reprinted London: Karnac Books, 1992].

Klein, M. (1932). The technique of analysis in puberty. In: *The Psycho-Analysis of Children* (pp. 80–94). London: Hogarth Press, 3rd edition, 1986.

Kohut, H. (1971). *The Analysis of the Self.* New York: International Universities Press.

Kramer, S. (1974). Episodes of severe Ego regression in the course of an adolescent analysis In: M. Harley (Ed.), *The Analyst and the Adolescent at Work* (pp. 190–231). New York: Quadrangle.

Ladame, F. (1991). L'adolescence, entre rêve et action. *Revue Française de Psychanalyse, 55*: 1491–1542.

Lagache, D. (1958). *Oeuvres complètes,* II. Paris: Presses Universitaires de France, 1977–1986.

Lampl-de Groot, J. (1960). On adolescence. *Psychoanalytic Study of the Child, 15*: 95–103.

Laplanche, J., & Pontalis J. B. (1967). *The Language of Psychoanalysis*. London: Hogarth Press, 1973. [Reprinted London: Karnac Books, 1988.]

Laufer, M. (1964). Ego ideal and pseudo ego ideal in adolescence. *Psychoanalytic Study of the Child, 19*: 196–221.

Laufer, M. (1968). The body image, the function of masturbation, and adolescence. *Psychoanalytic Study of the Child, 23*: 114–137.

Laufer, M. (1974). The analysis of an adolescent at risk. In: M. Harley (Ed.), *The Analyst and the Adolescent at Work* (pp. 269–296). New York: Quadrangle.

Laufer, M. (1975a). *Adolescent Disturbances and Breakdown*. London: Penguin Books.

Laufer, M. (1975b). Preventive intervention in adolescence. *Psychoanalytic Study of the Child, 30*: 511–528.

Laufer, M. (1996). De quelques préalables au travail psychanalytique avec des adolescents. *Adolescence, 14*: 239–245.

Laufer, M., & Laufer, E. (1984). *Adolescence and Developmental Breakdown. A Psychoanalytic View*. New Haven: Yale University Press. [Reprinted London: Karnac Books, 1995.]

Lebovici, S. (1980). L'expérience du psychanalyste chez l'enfant et chez l'adulte devant le modèle de la névrose infantile et de la névrose de transfert. *Revue Française de Psychanalyse, 44*: 733–857.

Lipschütz, A. (1919). *Die Pubertätsdrüse und ihre Wirkunge*. Bern.

Mahler, M. S. (1963). Thoughts about development and individuation. *Psychoanalytic Study of the Child, 8*: 307–324.

Mâle, P. (1982). La crise juvénile. In: *Oeuvres complètes I*. Paris: Payot.

Marty, F. (1996). Adolescence et puberté dans l'oeuvre de Freud. *Les Cahiers du Collège International de l'Adolescence, 1*: 83–97.

Noshpitz, J. D. (1957). Opening phase in the psychotherapy of adolescents with character disorders. *Bulletin of the Menninger Clinic, 21*: 153–164.

Nunberg, H., & Federn, E. (Eds.) (1962). *Minutes of the Vienna Psychoanalytic Society, Vol. I: 1906–1908*. New York: International Universities Press.

Nunberg, H. & Federn, E. (Eds.) (1967). *Minutes of the Vienna Psychoanalytic Society, Vol. 2: 1908–1910*. New York: International Universities Press.

Nunberg, H. & Federn, E. (Eds.) (1974). *Minutes of the Vienna Psychoana-*

lytic Society, Vol. 3: 1910–1911. New York: International Universities Press.

Nunberg, H., & Federn, E. (Eds.) (1975). *Minutes of the Vienna Psychoanalytic Society, Vol. 4: 1912–1918*. New York: International Universities Press.

Ouvry, O. (1996). Naissance du concept d'adolescence. *Les Cahiers du Collège International de l'Adolescence, 1*: 61–82.

Rank, O. (1909). *The Myth of the Birth of the Hero*, together with *The Trauma of Birth*. New York: Robert Brunner, 1952.

Rank, O. (1924). *The Trauma of Birth*, together with *The Myth of the Birth of the Hero*. New York: Robert Brunner, 1952.

Reich, A. (1954). Early identifications as archaic elements in the superego. *Journal of the American Psychoanalytic Association, 2*: 218–238.

Rieger, C. (1900). *Die Castration in rechtlich, socialer und vitaler Hinsicht*. Jena: G. Fischer.

Root, N. N. (1957). A neurosis in adolescence. *Psychoanalytic Study of the Child, 12*: 320–334.

Roussillon, R. (1995). La métapsychologie des processus et la transitionnalité. *Revue Française de Psychanalyse, 52*: 1352–1519.

Spiegel, L. A. (1951). A review of contributions to a psychoanalytic theory of adolescence: individual aspects. *Psychoanalytic Study of the Child, 6*: 375–393.

Tausk, V. (1919). On the origin of the "influencing machine" in schizophrenia. *Psychoanalytic Quarterly, 2* (1933): 519–556. [Reprinted in: R. Fliess (Ed.), *The Psycho-Analytic Reader* (pp. 31–64). London: Hogarth Press, 1950.]

Winnicott, D. W. (1961). Adolescence: struggling through the doldrums. In: *The Family and Individual Development* (pp. 79–87). London: Tavistock, 1965.

Winnicott, D. W. (1971). Contemporary concepts of adolescent development and their implications for higher education. In: *Playing and Reality* (pp. 138–150). London: Tavistock.

INDEX

www.ingramcontent.com/pod-product-compliance
Ingram Content Group UK Ltd.
Pitfield, Milton Keynes, MK11 3LW, UK
UKHW022202190926
475702UK00003B/157